ORGAN
DONOR

*A Dr. Beckett Campbell Medical Examiner
Thriller*

Book 1

Patrick Logan

Books by Patrick Logan

Detective Damien Drake

Book 1: Butterfly Kisses (feat. Chase Adams, Dr. Campbell)
Book 2: Cause of Death (feat. Chase Adams, Dr. Campbell)
Book 3: Download Murder (feat. Chase Adams, Dr. Campbell)
Book 4: Skeleton King (feat. Dr. Campbell)
Book 5: Human Traffic (feat. Dr. Campbell)
Book 6: Drug Lord: Part I
Book 7: Drug Lord: Part II

Chase Adams FBI Thrillers

Book 1: Frozen Stiff
Book 2: Shadow Suspect
Book 3: Drawing Dead
Book 4: Amber Alert
Book 4.5: Georgina's Story
Book 5: Dirty Money
Book 6: Devil's Den

Dr. Beckett Campbell Medical Thrillers

Book 0: Bitter End
Book 1: Organ Donor
Book 2: Injecting Faith (feat. Chase Adams, Tommy Wilde)

First Edition: March 2019

ORGAN DONOR

Prologue

DR. BECKETT CAMPBELL STOOD in the shadows, his eyes fixated on the taxicab as a large man in a white T-shirt stepped out. The man had shoulder-length brown hair that was pulled back into a greasy bun, and close-set eyes that were as dark as the night.

Beckett had seen him before.

He'd seen the man on TV over a year ago and then he'd seen him again on the news a few days prior after the judge had reluctantly declared that they had a hung jury.

A *second* hung jury.

Winston Trent was his name, and he would live the rest of his life as an accused, but never convicted, child murderer and rapist.

Twice he had been tried for the murder of nine-year-old Bentley Thomas, but both attempts to put him behind bars had failed. Beckett was a forensic pathologist and medical examiner and not a lawyer, but he knew enough about science to conclude that Winston was getting off on a technicality. A semen stain found at the crime scene was deemed inadmissible as it was stored incorrectly before a DNA profile had been generated—it had been placed in a mislabeled container.

It didn't matter that there was only a one-in-five-billion chance that the DNA belonged to anyone *but* Winston Trent, the defense argued. Or that the type of container was irrelevant and that the DNA wasn't tampered with or degraded. What the CSU tech had done was cast a shadow on the entire case, shooting reasonable doubt into the chain of command the way Winston had shot his load in the warehouse where Bentley's corpse had been discovered.

But Beckett wasn't bound by the same rules as the lawyers, the judge, or even the jurors; he had his own guiding principles, ones that superseded all other laws.

And he knew that Winston Trent was a guilty man. It wasn't just the sadistic grin plastered on his face as he taunted Bentley's family after the two mistrials. It was his eyes. His dark eyes were flat and even.

Eyes that Beckett recognized in himself when he stared in the mirror.

Beckett performed a cursory rundown of his own equipment and clothing as Winston made his way up the steps to his trailer. Beneath a black jogging suit, his body was covered in saran wrap to avoid leaving any of his own DNA at the scene. On top of his head he wore a balaclava that was rolled up, and in a gloved hand, he held a small leather case.

Although he didn't open the case, not just yet, he knew exactly what was inside. He knew because he'd checked a half-dozen times already.

Beckett had made some mistakes with the others—Craig Sloan, Donnie DiMarco, Ray Reynolds, Bob Bumacher, Boris Brackovich—but he was a quick study.

He wouldn't make the same mistakes again.

This time was going to be different.

Beckett waited until Winston slid the key into the trailer door before pulling a syringe from the case and hurrying across the street. He wasn't worried about being seen here; the people in this neighborhood loathed Winston Trent as much as any other and would turn a blind eye to anything that happened to him.

It was basic human psychology; if you wanted something to happen badly enough, you will accept your reasoning no matter how flawed when it eventually does occur.

If the gambler believes that his underwear is lucky before a big win, it was nearly impossible to convince them otherwise after the fact.

Someone as reprehensible as Winston Trent *must* abhor himself, so why wouldn't his death be a suicide?

Peering up at the sweat stains beneath Winston's arms and the dark V that extended down his back, Beckett spoke for the first time in several hours.

"Winston," he said simply.

The man opened the door and then turned. When he caught sight of Beckett, dressed all in black, a smile appeared on his thin lips.

"What the fuck you want?" he snapped. "I ain't givin' out no autographs."

With the hand holding the syringe still behind his back, Beckett took two steps up the stairs. When Winston responded by reaching inside the door, it was Beckett's turn to smile.

The man wouldn't find what he was looking for. In fact, if he turned around, not only would Winston not see his shotgun resting against the doorframe, but he might not even recognize the interior of his trailer.

Beckett had done some redecorating; when he'd come earlier in the day, the decor had not been to his liking.

He'd gone to the trouble of hanging images of Bentley Thomas's smiling face from pieces of thread that crisscrossed the interior of the trailer.

Beckett had also cleaned up a little; not because he'd wanted to, but because he needed to make room for his table and his tools.

"You killed that boy," Beckett said matter-of-factly.

Winston's grin became a sneer.

"That's not what the jury said," he snapped back. Winston was becoming visibly nervous now, reaching for a shotgun that wasn't there.

Beckett knew that he only had a few moments before Winston gave up and bolted inside, slamming the door in his face.

With an agility only afforded to him by his heightened state, Beckett bounded up the final three stairs until he was within inches of the foul-smelling Winston Trent.

"You better get off my property," Winston ordered. "Or you're—"

When the man's eyes flicked to the interior of the trailer, Beckett pounced. Catching the much bigger man by surprise, Winston stumbled over the lip of the doorway and fell backward.

Beckett landed on his chest and then drove the syringe into the soft skin on the side of his neck. Then he grabbed the man's chin and forced his head backward.

"Look around, Winston; you killed that boy—you killed Bentley Thomas. Just say it and I'll make this *less* painful than you deserve."

PART I

The Grand Opening

Chapter 1

"YOU'RE LATE," SUZAN CUTHBERT said out of the corner of her mouth.

Dr. Beckett Campbell wiped the sweat from his brow.

"Yeah, well, so long as *you're* not late, then I'm not all that worried," he shot back.

Suzan glared at him, but the lower half of her face gave her away; there was a hint of a smile forming on her pretty lips.

"You should—" she began, but Beckett elbowed her playfully in the ribs and lifted his chin towards the stage in front of them.

"C'mon, Suze, can't you see I'm trying to listen here?" he joked.

The truth was, this was the *last* place Beckett wanted to be right now. The opening of another hospital wing, the McEwing Transplant Unit, inaugurated by some douchebag with silver hair and deeply tanned skin who had likely never set foot in a public hospital in his entire life.

It didn't matter that Beckett himself had been elected to the board of directors for the new wing; he still didn't want to be here.

The man at the podium introduced himself as Sir — yes, *Sir,* as if he were a knight in shining armor — Francis England and looked to be between 45 and 55 years of age. Therefore, Beckett assumed that he was actually 102 and was being kept alive by a very specific cocktail of Botox, hair dye, and exogenous testosterone.

"Now, before I cut this here ribbon," Sir Douche began, "I would like to formally introduce two very proud members of the McEwing family, the late Peter McEwing's children, who also serve on the board of the McEwing Foundation. Please put your hands together and help me welcome Flo-Ann and Grant McEwing."

Jesus, the guy speaks like he's starring in a Monty Python flick, Beckett thought, then immediately regretted the opinion. *How dare I soil the Python name by thinking such filth?*

Sir England pressed his lips together and clapped with hands that looked like aged beef jerky.

Beckett shuddered and Suzan nudged him until he clapped along with the rest of the sheep.

Once he managed to peel his eyes off the spectacle that was Sir England, he realized that he knew Grant McEwing. Well, more precisely, Beckett knew *of* him. He had spent a month or two learning from the late Peter McEwin during his residency, and the man had talked at length about how bright his son was, how good a doctor he was going to make one day.

"Recognize Grant?" Suzan whispered as she continued to clap. "He's one of your residents this year."

Beckett's eyes focused on Grant's face, his shaved head, the narrow nose.

Then he raspberried his lips.

Nepotism at its finest.

"Lucky me."

Beckett's focus quickly shifted to Flo-Ann, a woman in her early twenties with short, blond hair cut bluntly just below her ears. She was wearing a Navy skirt that she picked at nearly constantly, pulling it away from her thighs, as she stepped forward. Grant moved with her, but he stayed behind his sister as she adjusted the microphone.

Flo-Ann cleared her throat before addressing the crowd.

"First of all, I would like to thank everybody involved with bringing my father's dream to light, including Sir England and the rest of the board of directors." Beckett did a small curtsy. "For those of you who don't know, Peter McEwing was my father. But he was more than just a great dad; Peter was also an accomplished transplant surgeon and it had been one of his dreams to one day open a brand new, state-of-the-art Transplant Unit right here in New York City. And you have made his dream come true."

Beckett raised an eyebrow. Although he didn't have the greatest memory under the best of circumstance, and spending just a few months with the man during rotations didn't leave an indelible mark, Beckett recalled that Peter McEwing was as boring as waiting in line at the Post Office.

But most doctors were, anyway; it was essentially part of the training. In fact, Beckett was debating starting a course that revolved around this very idea.

Doctor Etiquette 101: how to make a shit ton of money while being an asshole.

Maybe a course isn't the best idea, Beckett thought. *But a self-published book on Amazon? Shit, if a children's book about a homophobic bunny could get a bestseller tag, anything was possible.*

Flo-Ann looked as if she had more to say, but Sir England nudged her out of the way and commandeered the mic.

"Now for the official inauguration of The McEwing Transplant Unit!" he exclaimed. Someone from behind Sir England handed him a pair of comically large scissors. There was some confusion as to who would hold the scissors, but eventually all three of them—Grant, Flo-Ann, and Sir England—wrapped their hands on the plastic handle and together they cut the ribbon.

Beckett rolled his eyes. It was all ceremonial bullshit, which was as fake as Sir England's accent.

He looked over at Suzan.

"Hey, you want to get out of here?"

Suzan blinked.

"To prepare for the upcoming semester, I presume?"

Beckett rolled his eyes again.

"Oh, yeah, sure. We'll do something *very* responsible."

Suzan shrugged.

"It's not like you do any work, anyway," she replied. "Where would you be without me? On second thought, don't answer that—probably a ditch or an alley. By the way, a package came for you earlier—it's on your desk."

"What are the odds?" Beckett replied with a smirk. "I've got a package for you, too."

Chapter 2

"GOOD MORNING, DELORES," BECKETT said as he entered the hallway leading to his office with Suzan in tow.

The woman looked up from the newspaper she was reading and offered him a weak smile. She had wide, puffy cheeks, and a doughy expression that for some strange reason reminded Beckett of Oysters Rockefeller.

"Morning, Dr. Campbell," she replied.

Typically cheery to the point of curdling Beckett's stomach, her demure tone made him stop.

"Alright, Delores. Tell me what's wrong."

Delores pressed her lips together and handed the paper over to Beckett.

"What could be so—"

When his eyes fell on the inset mugshot, his heart skipped a beat.

Winston Trent, accused child killer, takes his own life, the headline read.

Beckett swallowed hard.

"Sickening, isn't it? Just doesn't seem fair that he gets off so easily," Delores said, but Beckett barely heard the woman.

His mind had transported elsewhere, and he suddenly found himself back in Winston's dilapidated trailer.

'You do this, and you're no better than me', Winston screamed as Beckett pressed the scalpel against the soft skin of his wrist. 'You hear that? You're no better than me!'

Beckett paused and he stared at the line of blood that seeped from the incision.

'I never said I was better than you, Winston. But you know who was better than both of us?'

'Don't do this, please,' Winston pleaded, tears in his eyes. *'I'm begging you.'*

'Little Bentley Thomas, that's who. He was better than both of us.'

"Looks like that asshole got what he deserved," Suzan offered.

Beckett shook his head and handed the paper back to Delores.

"I'm going to have to side with Suzan on this one; he most definitely got what he deserved."

Delores shook her head.

"But imagine what would have happened to him if he went to prison? A child rapist and murderer? *That* is what he deserved."

"Welp, happy Monday," Beckett said as he backed away from the desk. "Have a good one, Delores."

"You too, Dr. Campbell."

***

"Well? Are you going to open it?" Suzan asked.

Beckett looked at the large cardboard box on his desk.

"No, not with you here. What if it's some racy negligée from one of my other lovers?"

Suzan nearly choked on her iced coffee.

"Well, even if I can overlook your use of the disgusting term 'lovers,' I'd say that no one is willing to put up with your shit. Except for me… but that's only because I'm too young and naïve to know better."

Beckett nodded; she had a point.

"What the hell," he said as he tore the tape off the top of the box. Suzan was pretending not to be interested, but

Beckett knew better; she was far too focused on the forensic pathology course outline that she herself had created.

Turning the unboxing into a charade, Beckett started peeling the top back slowly while making exaggerated facial expressions, but when he saw what was inside, his brow furrowed.

"It's a little early for drinks, even for me," he said to himself as he stared at a white vinyl cooler.

He pulled it out and then used his elbow to push the cardboard box off to one side.

The cooler was cold to the touch.

Confused, Beckett frowned and unzipped the top.

"What the hell?" he whispered.

The cooler was cold because it was nearly filled to the top with dry ice. But this wasn't what gave Beckett pause, it was what was lying atop the dry ice that did that: a thick plastic bag adorned with a biohazard symbol. Inside the bag, which was filled with a peach-colored liquid, was something dark red roughly the size of a dinner plate.

"What is it?" Suzan asked, rising from the chair.

Beckett didn't answer; he was transfixed on the item in the bag. He was so focused on it, in fact, that he barely noticed a yellow piece of paper stuck to the side of the cooler.

He grabbed the bag with both hands and held it up to the light.

"Is that… is that what I think it is?" Suzan asked, trepidation creeping into her voice.

Beckett sloshed the bag around.

"It looks like someone thinks I've been drinking a little too much lately—it's a liver," he said matter-of-factly. It was then that Beckett noticed a second bag that had been buried beneath the first. He picked this one up, too. "It's been a while since I took an anatomy class, but I'm pretty sure this is a heart and this is a liver. The real question is, what the fuck are they doing on my desk?"

Chapter 3

"I CALLED THE TRANSPLANT department and they're not missing any organs," Suzan said, staring at the heart and liver in their respective biohazard bags.

"Well that's something you don't hear every day," Beckett grumbled. "You sure? I mean, with the new wing opening, maybe…"

Suzan shrugged.

"I called the transplant department, the morgue, even the lab—everyone I could think of. They aren't missing any organs, Beckett."

"Well, somebody sure as hell is."

Suzan leaned in close.

"You sure there's no requisition form in there?"

"Only this," Beckett said, grabbing the yellow note off the side of the vinyl cooler. "*Home is where the heart is.*"

Suzan raised an eyebrow.

"Really? Isn't that a country song? What the hell is this, Beckett? Some weird game between pathologists? A *whodunit* for organs?"

It was Beckett's turn to shrug; he had no clue what this was all about.

"Think you can do me a favor, Suze?" Beckett said as he put the note down and zipped the cooler closed. "Can you take the cooler to the new transplant wing? You know how people are with this shit… all defensive and whatnot. Nobody wants to admit that something as valuable as a heart and liver was misplaced. I bet if you take it in person, they'll give you some lame excuse, but in the end, they'll make sure that the heart finds a new home. Get it?"

Suzan didn't appreciate the joke and looked as if she were about to protest.

"Please, Suze."

"Fine," she replied. "But when I'm gone, you have to take a look at the course outline… make sure that everything you want the residents to learn this semester is on there."

Beckett smiled.

"It's a deal."

With that, Suzan picked the cooler up by the handle and left the office.

Only after she was gone and the door was closed behind her, did Beckett look at the note more closely.

There was something about it, something that was off… something that was *more* off than receiving a random heart and liver in an organ transplant cooler.

Even as Senior Medical Examiner for the state of New York, this was a new one for Beckett.

"Home is where the heart is," he read out loud. It was written in black ink in all capital letters. He flipped it over, expecting more, but that's all there was: HOME IS WHERE THE HEART IS. Beckett held the paper up to the light and noticed that even though the words were written with a soft marker—a Sharpie, maybe—there were indentations behind those letters, behind the words, as if someone had written on the pad with a pencil before tearing this sheet off.

Chewing the inside of his lip, Beckett went to his desk and scanned the piece of paper. After an image of the note appeared on his computer monitor, he went about enhancing the pencil indentations. He half expected it to be nonsense, a grocery list, perhaps, but anything might help him figure out who had sent the box.

He managed to delete *HOME IS WHERE THE HEART IS* and, by messing around with the contrast, words started to appear.

Beckett's breath suddenly caught in his throat and his heart thumped in his chest.

It wasn't nonsense, far from it: the indentations made a simple sentence, not that much unlike the message proclaimed in black ink.

And Beckett knew without a doubt that this message was intended for him and that the organs hadn't accidentally ended up on his desk.

Someone had sent them to him on purpose.

"I know what you are," Beckett whispered, his eyes locked on the computer screen.

Chapter 4

Beckett stared at the hidden message for a long while. And then, when he had committed it to memory—*I know what you are*—he messed around a little more in Photoshop to see if there were any other indentations.

There weren't.

With a hard swallow, Beckett deleted all of the images and then tucked the note into his pocket.

It was cryptic, it was vague, and yet Beckett knew what the anonymous writer meant.

I know what you are.

Out of habit, Beckett reached below his right arm and traced the tattooed lines that ran across his ribs. As he did, he repeated in his mind the names of the people that those lines represented.

Craig Sloan… Donnie DiMarco… Ray Reynolds… Bob Bumacher… Boris Brackovich… Winston Trent…

The phone on his desk buzzed and he startled. Seeing that it was Suzan, he picked it up and took a deep breath before answering.

"I don't know what to tell you, Beckett, but they're not missing any organs over here. In fact, they told me that during the transition to the new Unit, all transplants are taking place in Long Island. They called the Long Island transplant team for me, but they're not missing them, either."

Beckett chewed the inside of his lip as he mulled this over.

I know what you are.

"Shit," he said, trying to inject humor into his voice even though he was feeling none of it. "What do you want to do?

Take an ad out on Craigslist? *Hey, if anybody's missing a heart or a liver, give us a call.*"

He expected Suzan to laugh, but she didn't; the only reply was dead air.

"Suze? You still there?"

"Yeah, I'm here."

Her tone was strangely deadpan.

"I guess... I guess, bring the cooler to the lab? Ask them to perfuse the organs and keep them viable as long as possible."

"Okay," Suzan replied. "But what do you want me to say about them?"

"Tell them... tell them we're just waiting on some paperwork. And if they give you any trouble, tell them to call me."

Again, another hesitation.

"Okay, I'll take it to the lab. Are you sure that this isn't just a messed-up prank from one of your colleagues?"

Beckett thought about this for a moment. It wasn't impossible, of course, you had to be a special kind of weird to be a forensic pathologist, but the note, combined with the inauguration of the new transplant wing...

Beckett pictured Flo-Ann and Grant McEwing and the impeccably dressed Sir Francis England, their hands all gripping the comically oversized scissors.

"Yeah, I don't think so, but I'm gonna go see the venerable Sir Francis England myself. See what he has to say about all this."

"What about the course outline?"

"The what?"

"The outline," Suzan repeated. "You promised that if I chaperoned your organs around town, you'd read it over. But I'm guessing you haven't gotten around to it, have you?"

"Hellllll, no," Beckett said and then hung up the phone before Suzan could reply.

***

Beckett kept his hand on the note in his pocket as he walked down the hallway, ignoring those who milled about in lab coats. He was so focused on finding out where the organs had come from, that he didn't initially hear his name being called. In fact, he only stopped because someone reached for and grabbed his arm.

Beckett instinctively pulled away and his free hand curled into a fist.

"I'm sorry, I didn't mean to startle you," the man said.

"Then you shouldn't—" Beckett blinked. "Wait, it's you—from the ceremony. Grant McEwing."

Another coincidence, he thought glumly. *I don't like coincidences.*

For perhaps the only time in his life, Beckett wished he'd spent more time awake at the Board Meetings for the new transplant unit.

"What… what are you doing here?" Beckett asked.

"I just came to introduce myself, but I guess you know me already. I'll be starting as a pathology resident this semester."

Grant held out his hand as he said this and Beckett had to deliberately unclench his fist before shaking it. Grant's hand was clammy and his grip was that of a prepubescent girl.

"I also just wanted to say that I'm a big fan of yours and after I'm done with my residency, I want to be a medical examiner, too."

Beckett raised an eyebrow.

A fanboy?

It was clear that while Grant McEwing came from some decent stock, given that the transplant wing was named after his family and that Peter McEwing was a famed surgeon, he lacked something in terms of social graces and etiquette. And he was also just plain awkward.

"Why in the world would you want to do that?" Beckett asked. It was a rhetorical question, but, of course, Grant didn't pick up on this.

"Well, I guess I just like the idea of solving puzzles—the mystery aspect of it all."

Beckett chuckled.

"Then I suggest you stick to Nancy Drew and crosswords. Most of the time, I'm elbow deep in entrails, trying to figure out the last thing a person ate before they offed themselves. Trust me, kid, it just ain't all that interesting."

The two men stared at each other for several seconds with neither of them saying anything. Beckett knew that he should probably speak up, but he rather enjoyed seeing Grant squirm. If the man was uncomfortable in this situation, how in the world would he act when he was trying to figure out whose arm was whose after a three-car pileup?

But, alas, Beckett ran out of patience; besides, he had more pressing things to take care of.

"Well, it was great to meet you, Grant," Beckett said. "See you in class."

Grant nodded and started to walk away, his gait slow and awkward, much like the entire encounter.

Beckett watched the man go, grateful that Grant was destined to become a pathologist and hadn't chosen a discipline that—God forbid—required actual interaction with patients.

Chapter 5

"FRANCIS! *FRANCIS!*" BECKETT SHOUTED, waving a hand in the air.

As luck would have it, just as Beckett was walking toward the McEwing Transplant Unit, he caught sight of Sir Francis England heading out the back.

Another coincidence…

Francis had a cell phone pressed to his ear and was walking toward the rear door of a black Lincoln Navigator, which was held open by a no-nonsense looking man in a suit.

Now, who's the fanboy, Beckett thought as he hurried to catch up to Francis. He reached him just before the man lowered himself into the car.

"Francis!" Beckett said again. This time, he was positive that the man had heard him and yet the silver fox still didn't turn. "Hey, Frank!"

Beckett reached for Francis's shoulder, but the man in the suit holding the door blocked his path.

"I'm sorry," he began, placing a hand firmly on the center of Beckett's chest.

Beckett immediately swatted it away.

"You will be if you touch me again," he warned. The change in tone finally got Francis's attention.

"Yes?" the man asked, turning to face Beckett. "How can I help you?"

"I'm on the board of directors for the new transplant unit."

The man's expression never changed, although Beckett wasn't sure if this was because he was pumped so full of botulin or if he just didn't give a shit.

Francis's response confirmed the latter.

"And?"

Beckett fought back an insult.

"I just had a couple of questions for you."

"Be quick. I have several meetings to get to."

Oh, how I would love to throttle ye.

"Yeah, sure, I get it—cryogenics and all that. I was just wondering if you were missing a liver."

Francis's eyebrows moved upward or his forehead stretched—Beckett couldn't be sure which—but he was certain he had the man's attention now.

"Excuse me?"

"Yeah, I was just, uh, wondering if you lost a heart and liver. You see, they just wound up on my desk and I have no idea who they belong to."

Francis stared at Beckett for a good thirty seconds or so, clearly trying to figure out if he was joking or not.

Beckett remained stone-faced.

"Who did you say you were again?"

"I didn't. But this is no joke. Imagine what the media might say if they found out that on the day that the McEwing Transplant Unit opened, a heart and a liver went missing. I wonder how that would play out?"

Francis frowned.

If he was the person responsible for the organs ending up on Beckett's desk, then he wasn't taking any of the bait.

"I'm sorry, but I'm just a figurehead. If there's been some sort of mix-up, you're going to have to speak with the director… Dr. Aaron Singh. I have nothing to do with the daily operations."

"But I—"

Francis nodded to his driver and the man closed the door so suddenly that Beckett's T-shirt almost got caught in it.

"Fuck," he swore, leaping backward. He was still collecting himself when the driver peeled off. "You fucking asshole."

Beckett had wanted to throttle Francis earlier, but now he wanted to eviscerate the man.

Oh, I hope you're behind all this. I would love to cut you.

His fingertips started to tingle and it took several deep breaths before the feeling passed.

I know what you are.

As the Lincoln disappeared from sight, Beckett turned back to the transplant unit.

He couldn't believe that six months ago the area had just been an empty field. Now, after lightning-fast construction, an entire wing had been added on to the hospital. Made of whitewashed stone and colorful glass inserts, it extended approximately a hundred feet from the southern side of the building.

Above the entrance, written in large, block letters was the name: The Grant McEwing Transplant Unit.

For some reason, those letters, even though they were made of metal, reminded Beckett of the note written in black ink.

Home is where the heart is.

Beckett hurried to the entrance, only to find it locked. Frustrated, he pressed his thumb on the intercom beside the door.

A second later, a female voice answered.

"I'm sorry, but the Grant McEwing Transplant Unit won't be open until next week. For all related inquiries, please contact the Long Island Transplant Unit."

Beckett leaned away from the door and stared at the ribbon that had yet to be cleaned up.

Didn't they just have the grand opening a few hours ago?

"Yeah, I'm not a patient, I'm a doctor—Dr. Beckett Campbell. I need to talk to the director… to Dr. Aaron Singh."

There was a short pause, during which time Beckett suspected that the secretary or whoever the woman inside the tiny box was, searched for his name.

"Is he expecting you?"

Beckett chewed the inside of his lip and bit back a snide remark.

"No, I don't think so. Just let him know that I have some fresh organs I'd like to donate."

Chapter 6

"I'M SORRY, YOU SAID you were a forensic pathologist? So why are you asking about organ transplant?"

Beckett frowned. When the man in the sparkling white lab coat, clearly just moments ago removed from its packaging, walked down the hallway to greet him, Beckett realized that they'd met before. While he hadn't recognized the man's name—Dr. Aaron Singh—his face, the broad nose, the thick lips, jolted his memory. If it served him correctly, Beckett thought they'd even co-chaired a symposium a couple of years back. But while Beckett remembered Dr. Aaron Singh, it was clear that this wasn't reciprocated.

He sighed.

"Look, this is getting annoying; I have two organs and you run a transplant clinic. Let's just play nice and combine the two, what do you say?"

Aaron Singh was not known for his humor and he didn't disappoint.

"The fact remains," the director began flatly, "that we aren't missing any organs. And without a requisition sheet, I'm afraid they would just sit on the shelf and go to waste."

Beckett threw his hands in the air.

"All right then, whatever. I've done my due diligence here. Listen, if you ever need a heart or liver, you'll find one… in the lab, where I'm going to leave the meat to rot."

Aaron pressed his thick lips together.

"Dr. Campbell, I wish I could help, but I'm swamped trying to get this place up and running."

The man waved an arm about the hallway as if the plain surroundings were supposed to impress Beckett.

They didn't.

"Yeah, sure, I understand. I'll see you at the next board meeting, I expect that you'll be there, too?"

The comment piqued Aaron's interest and he squinted at Beckett for a moment before replying.

"You're not... wait you *are* on the board, aren't you?"

Wow, he's a bright one, Beckett thought. *I must have been sleeping when they put hiring him to a vote.*

"Sure am."

Dr. Singh's tone suddenly changed.

"Well, I'll tell you what," he began, his eyes darting about, "I'll ask one of my tech guys —"

Beckett slapped the man on the back and he stumbled forward awkwardly.

"No, that's all right. I'll have my people look into it. Just one question for you," Beckett said. "You think that if Dr. McEwing was still around that he'd want the organs? I'm just wondering, because, you know, I'm pretty sure he died from liver failure."

Dr. Singh shook his head and stared at Beckett with glassy eyes.

"Cancer. Look, I'm sorry Dr. Campbell, I really am. It's just so damn stressful trying to get this place up and running. I'm sure... I'm sure that the address for the delivery just got mixed up. Like I said, I'll contact one of my lab guys and see if they can track down where they're supposed to go. But right now... right now I have to go to another goddamn meeting."

The man held out his hand, but instead of shaking it, Beckett clapped Dr. Singh on the back again and offered his best fake smile.

"Don't worry about it, I'm sure I'll find someone in need," he said as he started down the hallway. And then, under his breath, he muttered, "Asshole."

Organs were more valuable than enriched plutonium and yet nobody seemed to want to have anything to do with them... or him.

Chapter 7

IF IT HADN'T BEEN for the hidden message in the note, Beckett would have washed his hands clean of the situation. After all, he'd already gone above and beyond.

But that note…

I know what you are.

Beckett resisted the urge to take the piece of paper out of his pocket and look at it again.

What I am, is fucking tired, he thought. This was followed by a stream of rationalizations, reasons why the pencil indentations weren't meant for him, that they were pure coincidence, that they were benign, unintentional, irrelevant.

But he knew better.

Beckett shook his head.

It was warm for mid-September and Beckett found himself sticking to the shade offered by the canopy of London Planes as he made his way back from the newly minted McEwing Transplant Unit to his office at NYU medical. He hadn't cared much for the sun before his trip to the Virgin Gorda, and now, after returning, he cared for it even less.

I know what you are…

A shudder ran up his spine despite the warm air and Beckett instinctively picked up his pace. In his office, he hoped to be alone, inundated by AC, so that he could think.

He had no such luck.

Suzan sat in his chair, her worn Converse sneakers on his desk. She tucked her short, blond hair behind her ears when Beckett entered and despite the half-scowl on her lips, she looked incredibly pretty at that moment. He knew, of course, that having a relationship with her was probably frowned

upon given that, while he wasn't technically her teacher—
Suzan Cuthbert was still a medical student—she was his *de
facto* TA.

Except Beckett didn't give a shit. He liked Suzan; he liked
the way that she kept him honest, the fact that she didn't put
up with his shit. It could be frustrating at times, but it was also
challenging in a way that his previous girlfriends, if you could
call them such, couldn't live up to.

Girlfriend… is that what she is now? Beckett thought with a
smirk. *Are we going steady? Should I give her my pin?*

"I'm not sure why you're smiling, because I'm not: you *still*
haven't signed off on the course outline."

Beckett rolled his eyes and swatted Suzan's feet off his
desk.

"That's Brazilian hardwood. Best you treat it with respect."

Suzan glanced under the desk.

"It's from Ikea."

"Via Brazil. Anyways, I'll look over the outline… I just
forgot."

"And I bet you forgot about tonight, too," Suzan said.

Beckett raised an eyebrow.

"Of course not… it's your birthday… and Mother's Day
and Valentine's Day," Beckett took a deep breath and spewed
out every holiday that he thought might hold relevance to… a
girlfriend. "Christmas, Hanukkah, Ramadan, Father's Day,
Independence Day, uhhh, Kwanza? Chrismukkah?"

This last one turned Suzan's frown into a grin.

"Ah, that's better. Did anyone ever tell you that you should
smile more? A pretty girl like you…"

Beckett knew that this particular comment grated Suzan,
but she was used to his jabs and didn't take the bait.

Instead, she reached for a folder on his desk and tossed it at him. Beckett caught it and inside found a single sheet of paper. On this paper were seven names, but he only recognized one of them: Grant McEwing.

Beckett shrugged.

"Yeah, the new residents. So, what?"

Again, the patented Suzan scowl.

"I swear to God, Beckett, you'd forget your penis if it weren't attached to your body."

"I'm not sure who would be more sad about that… me or you."

"Don't flatter yourself; half the time I can barely find the damn thing. Speaking of which, I think you should open this year's course with an hour-long lecture on micropenises. Teach what you know. What do you say?"

"I'd say that I'm in the market for a new TA. Willing to pay with smokes and beer. Must have clean, recent STD test."

"Touché," Suzan replied, rising from his chair.

As soon as it was vacated, Beckett plopped himself down in it. That was another thing about Suzan, he could just let go in front of her. *Relax.* He didn't have to pretend to be the all-healing doctor, the unfailing pathologist, crime fighter extraordinaire. He could be tired in front of her, he could be sad, in fact, he could almost be his *true* self.

Almost.

I know what you are.

Beckett shuddered and a look of concern crossed over Suzan's face.

"You okay? You haven't been yourself lately—haven't been yourself ever since you got back from the Virgin Gorda."

This wasn't true, of course; in fact, if anything, Beckett was *more* himself since returning.

"I'm just tired," he said. This wasn't a complete lie; his sleep had been pretty shitty ever since what had happened on the boat with Donnie DiMarco.

And before that with Craig Sloan.

"Well, sorry to break the news, but you're not going to get caught up on that sleep anytime soon. At least not tonight."

"Why? You got something special planned for me? A new outfit, maybe? A ball-gag? You know how much of a sucker I am for a good ball-gag."

Suzan shook her head.

"No, dumbass. I don't have something planned, you do."

Beckett, more confused than ever, held his hands out at his sides.

"*Non ho capito una parola, Mademoiselle,*" he said with a smile.

"Classes start tomorrow, Beckett. Which makes tonight, hazing night."

Chapter 8

IT WASN'T *TECHNICALLY* HAZING night. Hazing went out of style and fashion when some 'roided up football player decided it would be a hoot to ram a broomstick up a couple of rookie's colons.

Not Beckett's idea of fun, and evidently not the rookie who pressed charges, either.

So, it wasn't *hazing* night. It was… *orientation evening*.

And while to an outsider, it might just look like a night of drinking and debauchery—and it mostly was—Beckett had a method to his madness.

Either that or his madness had a method.

He could never tell the difference.

"A quick toast," Beckett proclaimed, raising a shot glass filled to the brim with tequila. His voice could barely be heard over the music, and he motioned for the bartender to turn it down a few notches.

The man, a good friend of Beckett's, obliged.

"A quick toast," he repeated, louder this time. The eyes of his soon-to-be residents, as well as Suzan's, all focused on him. Their faces were a mixture of confusion and apprehension; like last year, and the year before that, these greenhorns didn't know what to make of the young forensic pathologist with bleach-blond hair and tattoos covering his chest and arms. A man who liked to drink tequila straight from the bottle, or in this case, from a shot glass. But that was partly the point; Beckett wanted to show them that their biases and preconceptions were just tricks that the brain used to simplify a complicated world.

But that didn't mean that they were accurate. And in the field of forensic pathology, an inaccurate cause of death might result in somebody ending up behind bars for the rest of their lives.

And it was also about drinking.

"This is no test," Beckett continued. "Tonight is going to be one of the last nights that you'll have the freedom to go all out, to indulge in whatever your heart desires. I recommend that you take advantage of this, that you party like it's nineteen ninety-nine."

Beckett regretted saying this last part—he wasn't sure that half the people in the room were alive in nineteen ninety-nine, let alone know what the hell he was talking about. Still, he tilted his shot glass and said, "So drink up, and I look forward to seeing everyone in class tomorrow."

With that, Beckett glanced over at Suzan and she raised her own shot glass in the air. They drank in unison.

When he was done, Beckett slapped his hands together and waved the bartender over for a second time. Leaning in close, he whispered in the man's ear and the bartender pulled back, a smile on his face.

Then he ducked below the bar, only to reappear a moment later with an entire bottle of Patron and nine clean shot glasses at the ready. The bartender cracked the bottle and filled the glasses in one pour.

"You guys better drink up, because tonight is on the good doctor," the bartender exclaimed before blasting the music again.

Beckett held his hands up and a small and somewhat confused cheer rippled through the crowd.

"Beckett, you *are* the man," he said, taking another shot glass and downing it. "And you've earned a few drinks."

***

Beckett slumped into a booth and wiped the sweat from his brow. He knew that his face had turned red as it often did when he drank, but he didn't care. Like his residents, this would be one last time for him to let loose as well.

"You having a good time, Suze?" he asked. Suzan was one of the few people in the bar who appeared relatively sober, which was something considering it was coming up on 2 a.m.

"Oh, just peachy," she replied. Only then did Beckett notice an open three-ringed binder in front of her. He reached out and grabbed it before Suzan could react, and then he started to read.

"Graves' disease? Seriously? You have to study something this easy?"

"Easy for you," Suzan shot back. When she reached for the binder, Beckett let her take it back.

"Easy for everyone. Go on, ask me anything."

Suzan closed the binder and rested a hand on top.

"Okay, fine. What's your natural hair color?"

Beckett chuckled.

"This is a wig—I'm bald. Ask me about Graves'."

He could tell by the expression on her face that she didn't like when he did this, when he showed off, but Beckett was feeling pretty good about himself and the alcohol had loosened his tongue.

"Fine, I'll just tell you then. Graves' disease is an autoimmune disease that primarily affects the thyroid. It occurs in roughly half a percent of the male population, three percent in women, and is often associated with the following symptoms: tremors, weight loss, muscle wasting, goiter development, and tachycardia. The most common observable sign is a bulging of the eyes. You want me to continue?"

Suzan shook her head.

"No."

"Seriously, I don't mind. The most common cause of hyperthyroidism, Graves' disease results from thyroid stimulating immunoglobulins that bind to the TSH receptor. This causes secretion of T4 and T3 by the thyroid, as a result… can I help you with something?"

Suzan raised an eyebrow, but then Beckett turned around to address the two men who had approached from behind. He recognized one as Grant McEwing and the other as a resident named Pedro or Pablo or something of the like.

The men were startled that Beckett had noticed them, but the truth was he knew that they were there all along.

He'd only hoped that they would walk away without him having to address them. Clearly, that wasn't happening.

"Well? Are you just gonna stare at my pretty face or do you have a pressing question that you want to ask?"

Grant blushed, but the other man, imbued with liquid courage, cleared his throat.

"Me and a couple of the guys… you see, we have this bet… about your finger."

While no actual question had been posed, Beckett was a doctor and not a lawyer.

He decided to play along.

"This little thing?" he said, raising his right hand and wagging the middle finger. It was only two thirds as long as the others, ending just before the final knuckle in a flap of smooth skin.

"Lawnmower accident when I was younger. Fought with two reciprocating metal blades and lost."

Pablo or whatever his name was smiled and looked at Grant. Then he slapped the man roughly on the back.

"Told you," he exclaimed. "I told you... now you owe me a drink."

Grant turned to look at Beckett for support.

"No—no he doesn't," Beckett said. "Not tonight, anyway. Tonight's on me. Now move along and let me enjoy my drink, would you?"

When they were alone again, Beckett turned back to Suzan and was surprised to see that she was shaking her head.

"Lawnmower accident? Really?"

Beckett shrugged.

"A man has got to have some secrets. Speaking of which, I've got something to show you..."

Chapter 9

BECKETT SIGHED AND STARED up at the ceiling, which was bathed in a bluish glow from the moonlight that filtered in through the open window. It had been a hot night, unseasonably so, and he was sweating profusely.

It was also the alcohol—he could smell it coming out of his pores.

Suzan rose and went to the bathroom and, when she returned, she'd thrown on one of Beckett's T-shirts. Without saying a word, she curled up beside him and rested her head on his bare chest. For several minutes they just lay there, breathing in unison in the near darkness.

Beckett liked times like these, times when he didn't feel the need to fill the emptiness with speech. Even though he spent most of his days among the dead learning their secrets, his mind was always working, always trying to put together pieces of a rounded puzzle. Lying in bed beside Suzan was one of the few times that his mind went quiet.

It was as if everything he'd done over the past year or so, everything that had happened to him, was irrelevant. The only thing that mattered right now was that he was here, with her.

Beckett expected that Suzan felt the same way, as she too refrained from speaking.

Instead, she traced the tattoos on his chest, the bull on one pec, the Celtic symbol on the other, before moving her hand along the side of his body. Beckett's hands were above his head now, fingers interlaced, and when Suzan brushed against his newest tattoo, he flinched a little.

It was still raw and red.

Suzan propped herself up on one elbow and started to trace the two-inch lines that ran across his ribs. There were six of them now, the most recent of which he'd made less than two days ago.

"You ever gonna tell me why you gave yourself these tattoos?" she asked softly.

Beckett closed his eyes.

"They are a reminder," he replied. "Every one of my tattoos is a reminder of a specific point in my life."

It was a fairly generic comment and if it were anybody else but Suzan lying beside him, they might've gone for it. Suzan was much like him in that respect; he could tell her something, and she might accept it, but that wasn't enough. She needed more, she needed facts, details.

"But these lines... what do they represent?"

Beckett squeezed his eyes closed even tighter and hoped that Suzan didn't catch the strained expression on his face.

As she ran her fingers gently across each of the individual lines, Beckett started repeating the names of his victims in his head. It was something he did often on his own, but this was the first time that anybody else other than himself had touched these tattoos.

Craig Sloan... Donnie DiMarco... Ray Reynolds... Bob Bumacher... Boris Brackovich... Winston Trent...

The silence that ensued stretched for a good minute before Suzan addressed him again.

"Are you sleeping?"

Beckett shook his head but refrained from answering. Suzan snaked her hand up behind Beckett's head and started to massage his nub of a missing finger.

"Why do you lie to people when they ask about what happened to your finger?"

Beckett realized that Suzan's words were slurred and finally understood that she had drunk a little more than usual. Unlike him, she wasn't much of a drinker and the three or four shots of tequila must have gone right to her head.

Or her tongue, as it were.

"I told you, a man needs some secrets."

Another pause, only shorter this time.

"You don't need to keep secrets from me, Beckett. You can tell me anything."

Beckett drew a deep breath in through his nose and exhaled slowly.

"There are some things…" he paused, realizing that Suzan was now snoring softly on his chest. "There are some things about me that even you wouldn't understand. That *I* don't even understand."

In a matter of minutes, Beckett was snoring along with Suzan.

Chapter 10

"IN FRONT OF EACH of you, there is a body," Beckett said, his words echoing up and down the morgue. "On the tray beside the cadavers, you have all the tools that you need to come up with the cause of death. I will tell you straight up that not all of these people died from malicious causes, but some most definitely did. You have two hours to come up with the correct cause of death—this is your first test. It will set the stage for this entire year. The fact is, all of you either excelled in medical school, crushed your interviews, or your parents were rich enough to buy your way into a program you didn't earn. But I don't care—I don't care about any of that. The only thing that I care about is that you *are* here. And with that come certain expectations."

Beckett let his eyes drift over the residents, noting their pale faces and their messy or disheveled hair, the lack of makeup worn by the two women in the class. Eventually, his eyes fell on Grant McEwing, who looked particularly rough this morning, with dark circles beneath his bloodshot eyes.

I guess it also helps to have an entire transplant unit named after your family. That usually helps, Beckett thought.

He cleared his throat and continued.

"Up to this point in your schooling, you were likely forced to work alone, unable to speak to your colleagues or even use the Internet during tests. That's complete and utter bullshit. Your colleagues are a great asset and the Internet is perhaps man's greatest invention. What matters, what *really* matters, is coming up with the correct diagnosis or, in this case, the cause of death."

Beckett wasn't surprised by the chorus of raised eyebrows. In fact, he expected it.

"This isn't a joke... you can, and should, get started. You only have an hour and a half left."

One of the residents started to protest, but Beckett held up his hand.

"This is my class, which means my rules. Now get going."

With that, Beckett took a seat behind the desk off to one side and put his feet up. Then he grabbed his Styrofoam cup and started to sip the bitter sludge that passed as coffee nowadays. At first, none of the residents did anything; they just stood there, dumbfounded. Eventually, Maria Townsend, a rail-thin, birdlike creature, pulled back the sheet that covered the gurney in front of her. Beneath was a naked corpse of a man who was 350 pounds if he was an ounce. His wide face was blue and his body was covered in coarse hair that might've convinced Velcro to issue a cease and desist for patent infringement.

Upon seeing the corpse, Maria gagged. Beckett watched her curiously to see if she would recover, but she didn't. Her entire body shuddered and then she ran to the waste bin where she unloaded the contents of her stomach, which, based on the smell, was predominantly tequila.

Beckett spotted Pablo gagging out of the corner of his eye even though he hadn't pulled back the sheet on his cadaver yet. A moment later, the man joined Maria.

Vomiting in stereo was more than twice as bad, he realized.

"If you're going to be sick, be sick. I don't care," Beckett said with a chuckle. "Get your fellow residents a glass of water, some electrolytes, hook 'em up with an IV. We're not enemies here—you aren't in competition. That being said, you only have an hour and a quarter left. Better do *something*."

The haze of the alcohol from the night before slowly started to fade and the room was suddenly abuzz with sounds. There were people talking and there were others performing autopsies in near silence; the residents were indeed doing *something*. When he saw Grant McEwing cracking open the ribcage of his cadaver, his thoughts turned to what was behind those spoke-like bones, predominantly the heart.

Beckett had heard nothing about the organs that he'd instructed Suzan to take to the lab and found himself wondering where they had ended up. He also thought about the note.

I know what you are.

He shook his head and turned to his computer, distracting himself with boring housekeeping items: declining offers to publish in this predatory journal or that one, telling desperate wannabe residents that they were SOL.

Making sure his YouPorn subscription was up-to-date.

When he was done, Beckett checked his watch and realized that 40 minutes had passed since he first addressed his new residents.

He cleared his throat loudly to get their attention before speaking.

"I don't hear enough talking between you guys, so what I want you to do now is something I like to call musical cadavers, minus the music. Move one body to your right and start working on that cadaver. You guys are like a fraternity here—oops, I mean sorority, uhh, mixed-ority... *zimority?*— anyways, your success is predicated on you being able to help your fellow resident. And that's what I want you to do now. *Help.* Hive mind, people."

Maria, who had since returned to her cadaver and with a trembling hand was trying to sift through the thick blanket of yellow fat covering the man's organs, raised her gaze. Beckett almost laughed when he saw the sting of hatred in her eyes.

"Is that why you took us all out last night and got us drunk?" she asked, venom on her tongue. "Because we're supposed to be part of some sort of archaic Greek institution?"

Now Beckett did laugh. Normally he wouldn't be baited so easily, but seeing as this was the first class, he felt the need to explain.

"Feisty, *ooo*, I like that. But, no, that's not the reason. It was an eye-opener. You guys must have heard stories about residents working sixteen, eighteen, even twenty-hour shifts without even a single break to pinch a loaf. That's bullshit. You wanna know what causes physicians to make more mistakes than alcohol or drugs combined? Lack of sleep—I bet even you overachievers didn't know that. The irony is that a patient who smells alcohol on his surgeon's breath would never think twice about rescheduling their surgery. But a doctor who can barely keep his eyes open? That's the real danger. The thing you should ask your doctor before going under is how much sleep they had the night before.

"This whole idea of residents working double or triple shifts boils down to a single man: William Hallstead. Commonly known as the father of medical residency in the United States, William Hallstead was notorious for working long hours without seeming to tire. But our friend Bill had a secret. His secret was *cocaine*. Yes, children, the wonderful white powder that your mom said was just flour when you caught her rubbing her gums in front of her vanity. Back then, in the late eighteen-hundreds, cocaine was commonly used in surgery for its analgesic and anesthetic properties. Bill was quite fond of the powder and often tested it on himself for a variety of situations. This helped him work insanely long hours, and he expected others to do the same. To deal with his addiction—" Beckett stopped speaking when the door to the morgue opened and a startled looking Suzan poked her head in.

"You doing the whole coked-up Bill routine?" she asked. "Did he get to the part where they treated his cocaine addiction with Morphine?"

"Suzan! How dare you steal the punch line!" Beckett mocked, rising to his feet. "You guys keep working, I'll be back in a few," he told his residents. "And, before you ask, no you can't use cocaine. At least not during the test."

Despite Suzan's joke, when he made his way over to her, Beckett saw that she was paler than usual.

"What is it? What's up?"

Suzan swallowed hard.

"You've got another one… there's another package on your desk, Beckett."

Chapter 11

"**YOU'VE GOT TO BE** shitting me."

Beckett stood in the doorway of his office staring at the cardboard box on his desk. It was roughly the same size as the first one, and it was sealed up tight with clear tape.

"You're sure nobody saw this being delivered?" he asked Suzan who tentatively entered the room behind him.

She shook her head.

"I asked Delores and she said she didn't see anybody. It wasn't delivered by internal mail either and there are no stamps on it. I'm guessing someone just snuck in and hand-delivered it before anyone was at their desk."

Beckett stared at the box for several moments before actually making his way over toward it.

He could've overlooked the first delivery, racked that one up to being a mistake that his name had been slapped on by accident. He *might've* even been able to forget about the cryptic note. But this... a second delivery in as many days, that was more difficult to rationalize.

I know what you are.

Shaking his head, Beckett walked over to the box and reached for the frayed end of the tape. He was about to pull it back when Suzan laid her hand gently on his wrist.

"You think... you think that's a good idea?" she asked. Beckett looked at her, his brow furrowing.

"What do you mean?"

"I mean... maybe you shouldn't open it. Maybe we should get someone else to come and take a look at it."

"Someone else?"

Suzan lowered her eyes as she spoke.

"Yeah, like the police."

Beckett bit the inside of his lip. The last thing he wanted to do was get the police involved in *anything* that he did, given what happened last time. Most of his status as the Senior Medical Examiner and as the head of the forensic pathology program at the University had been reinstated after his "vacation," but Beckett was no idiot; he knew that others didn't appreciate his unconventional style.

The old guard wanted him gone. They wanted to protect their secrets, the recipe for the potion that kept people like Sir Francis England alive.

Beckett shook his head and then tore the tape off with one hard yank.

"*Yeaaah*, that's not happening."

Inside the box was a white vinyl cooler emblazoned with the words "Human Organ for Transplant" written in red on the side. It was the same style of cooler that the previous organs had been delivered in. With trepidation, Beckett started to unzip the top but, as before, Suzan's hand came down on his, halting his progress.

"You sure about this, Beckett?"

Beckett looked at her then, trying to figure out what she was getting at. Suzan knew that he was no saint, she knew what happened to his finger and what happened to Craig Sloan. And as far as he could tell, Suzan understood why he'd done what he had. After all, Craig had kidnapped her and if it hadn't been for Drake and himself, Suzan most likely would've burned alive inside that house.

And yet, there was something in her eyes, something that made Beckett think back to last night's questions about the tattoos, her odd statement that he could tell her anything that gave him pause.

I know what you are.

For a split second, Beckett considered that it might have been *her* who had written the note.

But then he shook his head. That was ridiculous.

Beckett gently brushed her hand away and then opened the cooler.

Inside, sitting in a bag of liquid atop pellets of dry ice, was an organ about the size of his fist.

"A heart," he heard Suzan whisper.

Beckett nodded in agreement. It was clearly a heart — a human heart, by the looks of it.

But Beckett wasn't focused on the heart, he was searching for another note. He found the yellow paper pressed against the side of the vinyl cooler, squeezed between the cardboard. Rather than pull it out, however, he turned to Suzan.

"Think you can do me a favor?"

Suzan nodded.

"Mind heading back to pathology to see if they're missing a heart? And can you please see what the lab is doing with yesterday's package?"

Suzan stared at him curiously for a moment and Beckett thought maybe that he had pushed her too far, that he was treating her now as a secretary and not a TA, but eventually, she nodded.

"What about you? What are you going to do?"

Beckett turned his eyes back to the yellow sheet of paper before answering.

"I'm thinking about opening up a shop: *Beckett's Bonafide Organs*. Probably pays better than this shit."

Chapter 12

BECKETT STARED AT THE note in his shaking hand. Written in black ink on the same yellow paper, the message was equally as simple as it was cryptic: *To live is to die.*

Beckett felt a strong urge to scrunch up the piece of paper and toss it in the garbage—pretend that it never existed. He also considered, albeit briefly, taking Suzan's advice and calling the police.

But he couldn't do that.

Whoever was sending these organs knew something about Beckett, something that he hadn't shared with anybody, not even Suzan.

With a frustrated grunt, Beckett held the note up to the light. There, beneath the black ink, were the familiar pencil indentations.

"Fuck," he grumbled as he lowered the paper onto the scanner. It took less than a minute for the image to appear on the screen and half that long for him to perform the same simple manipulations in Photoshop that he had with the other note. And like a magic 8-ball coming to rest, a message appeared.

I know what you did.

Beckett slammed his hand down on the desk.

No, the deliveries weren't the result of a drunken UPS courier—they had been sent to him on purpose.

What that purpose was, however, was still a mystery.

Beckett normally liked puzzles; this was, in fact, one of the reasons he'd gone into forensic pathology in the first place. But like the infuriating sudoku games in the *Saturday Times*, this was one that he didn't care for.

If this person really knows what I did… if they really know what my tattoos stand for, why not just go to the cops? Why send me hidden messages and goddamn body parts?

Beckett scowled.

The only reason that he could think of is that the mystery person wanted something.

But what?

Sure, Beckett had money, but not *that* much money. Besides, there was no indication of any sort of ransom.

He threw his hands up.

"Who are you? And what the hell do you want from me?"

The only answer was his own labored breathing.

Worried that Suzan would return shortly, Beckett took several deep breaths to calm himself and then deleted the image from his computer. Then he withdrew the first note from the top drawer of his desk. A brief comparison confirmed that they were indeed from the same person, but other than that, they provided no clues to their origin.

He put them both back in the drawer and was in the process of closing it when his phone buzzed. The noise was so startling that he slammed the drawer on his hand.

Only, he felt no pain.

His hand should have been throbbing, but when he looked down, he saw that the only finger that had been in jeopardy was his middle finger—the one that was missing.

Lawnmower accident…

Beckett lived in New York City for Christ's sake; nobody had a lawn, let alone a lawnmower. The truth was, he'd been abducted by some cult who called themselves the Church of Liberation. *They* were the ones who had cut off his fucking finger and were intent on making him one of their final victims. In the end, Beckett had made the leader of the cult, Ray Reynolds, one of *his*.

Without thinking, Beckett brought his hand to his ribs and traced his tattoos through his T-shirt.

Then he shook his head and looked down at his phone.

You keep acting like a fucking dope fiend, and Mr. Organ Donor won't be the only one who knows what you did... and who you are, he scolded himself.

He expected—and hoped—that the caller was Suzan, but when he looked at his phone, the message was from a number he didn't recognize.

I know the cause of death.

The sight of another cryptic message made his blood boil and, without thinking, Beckett dialed the number.

When a male voice answered, Beckett didn't wait for him to finish saying hello before he shouted into the phone.

"What the hell do you want from me? Why did you send me this shit?"

There was a short pause, and then he heard the man on the other end clear his throat.

"Dr. Campbell? It's Grant... I just wanted to let you know that we've figured out the cause of death."

Beckett inhaled sharply.

Grant? Who the hell is Grant?

"The cause of—" Beckett stopped midsentence.

Grant McEwing.

He'd completely forgotten about his residents back in the morgue. He took a deep breath.

"Shit, okay, everyone's done?"

There was another short pause before Grant replied.

"We think... we think we got them all. There's one that we're not so sure about and there's—"

"Yeah, I'll be there soon. Nobody leaves until I get there."

With that, Beckett ended the call and focused on the heart resting on the dry ice.

I know what you are… I know what you did…

Well, Beckett thought, his anger building again, *I don't know who or what* you *are, but I know what* you *did—and when I find you, you're going to regret this.*

When it came to the dead, Beckett liked a good mystery as much as the next forensic pathologist. But when it came to the living, it wasn't a puzzle so much as a hunt.

A hunt for a killer who needed to pay for what they'd done.

Chapter 13

"ALL RIGHT, STUDENTS. LET'S get this over with—I've got shit to do," Beckett said as he stormed into the morgue.

He was happy to see that Maria and Pablo appeared to have overcome their illnesses, and the rest were more sprightly than they had been just an hour ago.

Ah, the healing power of learning.

Mostly, Beckett was just happy for the distraction from other, more pressing matters.

"All right, I'm going to start from left to right. First up, Taylor: what's your cadaver's cause of death?" Beckett asked as he made his way over to a man with shoulder-length blond hair that had been tied up into a bun. The resident was hovering over the body of a nude woman who looked to be in her 80s. "Come on, everyone, gather around."

Beckett waited for everyone to do as he'd asked, and when they were all surrounding the corpse, he turned to Taylor again.

"Taylor?"

"It's Trevor," the man replied. Beckett just blinked at him, and eventually, the resident continued. "My cadaver is an eighty-year-old woman who appears to have died three or four days ago. I think—"

Beckett snapped his fingers.

"I asked for the cause of death, not the obituary. Let's get this show on the road."

Trevor's face reddened and he lowered his gaze.

"Based on the excess cranial pressure and the sheer volume of clotted blood on the brain, she died from hemorrhage due to an aneurysm."

"And why did you initially assume an aneurysm, Taylor? Tell me you didn't dull my bone saw just on a hunch."

The man used a pair of tweezers to lift the woman's eyelids.

"Her eyelids were drooped and the bleeding in her brain was so massive that blood leaked into the orbit through the sphenoid bone."

Beckett nodded.

"Good—you are correct. Now onto the next."

Beckett strode over to the second cadaver, the morbidly obese man covered in coarse hair that had initially been given to Maria.

"And whose corpse is this?"

The man's chest had been opened with a Y-incision and his rib cage spread wide, revealing his internal organs.

"This was mine," Grant McEwing said and Beckett encouraged the man to continue.

"Our man died from acute hepatic failure likely due to cirrhosis from excess alcohol consumption and/or fat consumption."

Beckett's eyes drifted to the pale pink liver that was enlarged and covered in ribbons of yellow fat.

"Good, now—"

Beckett leveled his eyes at Grant McEwing and he observed the man closely.

What are the odds that they open the McEwing Transplant Unit on the same day that Grant McEwing starts his residency? To top it off, I get a liver delivered to my office, and his cadaver just happens to die of liver failure?

It was all one hell of a coincidence, one that Beckett intended to put to the test.

"Why did you choose liver failure and not heart disease?" Beckett said, pointing at the enlarged heart which was also covered in yellow fat. "How do you know he didn't die of coronary artery disease? After all, *home is where the heart is*."

Beckett focused on Grant when he said this last part, but the man remained stone-faced. Some of the other students gave him a strange look, but Grant seemed unperturbed.

"Well," Grant continued. "This man would've undoubtedly died from coronary heart disease eventually given the plaque buildup in his arteries, but his liver gave out first. My cadaver had severe ascites and swelling of the lower limbs. He also had a tremendous amount of scarring around the hepatic artery. To be sure, I removed the heart and found that while the intima of all major arteries and veins were thickened, none of the lumens were occluded."

Beckett quieted Grant by waving his hand.

Right, you passed the test... both of them.

Beckett had more questions but feared drawing too much attention or, worse, having his interest misinterpreted as a sort of favoritism.

"Okay, let's keep moving."

The next body was that of a man who had died from blunt force trauma to the skull, which had caused skull fragments to puncture his brain and cause bleeding. Cadaver four was a woman who had died from advanced lung cancer that had spread to several of her organs. The students got both of these two correct, but when Beckett approached the next body, the fifth of eight, he immediately knew that this was the one that they were having trouble with.

This came as no surprise; the residents never got this one right.

"All right, whose is this?"

A nervous-looking man with a patchy beard and oversize spectacles spoke up.

"I don't know the name; there was no—"

Beckett rolled his eyes.

"Not who the victim is, but which resident had this body. And, judging by the way it looks like you crapped your pants, I'm guessing it's yours. Now, tell me what you've got."

The man cleared his throat and kept his eyes locked on the woman's corpse in front of them as he continued.

"Well, I think she drowned… clearly, her hands are the way they are because she'd been submerged for some time," the man said. As he spoke, he lifted the woman's forearm. The skin on her hand was wrinkled and shifted awkwardly like a loose condom.

She had washerwoman hands, an extreme form of pruning that occurred when bodies were submerged for a prolonged period of time after death.

"And? Did she drown? Your confidence is overwhelming, by the way."

The man hesitated before answering.

"I—I'm not sure. Clearly, she was in the water after death, but I can't conclude that she drowned."

"Why not?"

The resident indicated dark bruising on the woman's back.

"The settling of blood… if she drowned, I would expect for her to float belly up. That would cause lividity to form in her back, not her stomach."

"Only partly right. After drowning, most bodies sink, but once the bacteria in their stomach and guts start to party they rise to the surface. The limbs rotate downward, which effectively spin the body so that it rises with the back to the surface. But in these cases, the head hangs down and lividity and blood pooling often occur in the neck and face, not the stomach *or* the back."

Beckett grabbed a scalpel and pressed down on the exposed lungs.

"See that? If she drowned, there would be evidence of significant pulmonary edema. You know when you're wearing your best loafers and you step in a puddle? That squishy sound that happens with every step? That's what her lungs would be like if she drowned. So, if that wasn't the cause of death, what was?"

The smile now gone from patchy beard's face, he looked to his colleagues for support. When no one stepped forward, Beckett grew frustrated.

"Look, I already told you guys this isn't like medical school. You're not competing with each other, you're here to determine the cause of death. So, help poopy pants out here… how did this woman die?"

Eventually, Grant McEwing stepped forward.

"There is hemorrhaging around the eyes," he said softly.

"Speak up, man! There are no secrets here."

Except for maybe one…

Grant cleared his throat and when he spoke again, his voice was loud and clear.

"There is petechial hemorrhaging around her eyes, suggesting that she's been strangled. I also noticed, even though we didn't dissect her throat, some swelling there, which is consistent with strangulation."

Beckett tilted his head and observed the woman's pallid neck.

"Minimal swelling and bruising… what you are seeing is more likely a result of a hyoid bone fracture, which is jutting out. Congratulations, the cause of death is indeed strangulation."

He offered Grant a curt nod and let his eyes linger for a moment longer. If it was Grant who was, for some fucked-up reason, sending him these mysterious organs, he had a poker face that would give Chase Adams a run for her money.

"All right, onto the next."

It took less than 10 minutes to finish with the remaining corpses, and Beckett was surprised to see that they'd guessed each cause of death correctly.

"Alright, that's it for the day. Go home and get some rest or have a drink. Just no coke. See you back here tomorrow morning."

"That's it?" Maria asked. "It's not even eleven yet."

Beckett shrugged.

"Rest is super important. Rest, and a breath mint, Maria. Just a tip."

Chapter 14

BECKETT LEFT THE MORGUE and rushed back to his office. He was surprised that Suzan wasn't there but had more pressing matters to deal with. Even as his residents were telling him about their cadaver's cause of death, his mind had been elsewhere, trying to come up with a way to figure out who the hell was sending him the organs and cryptic messages.

Once in his office, his attention returned to the heart in the organ transplant cooler. It was impossible to know when it had been removed, but it looked healthy enough. Yet the time between removal and viability for a heart transplant was in the order of six hours or less, and it had already been sitting on his desk for three or four.

He didn't want to get anyone involved—not the cops, not the hospital—but Beckett *was* a doctor, and he wasn't oblivious as to just how valuable these things were.

"Shit," he swore. Then, against his better judgment, he grabbed his cell phone and scrolled through his contacts until he reached 'Lab Guy.'

A scratchy voice answered on the first ring.

"Lab Guy?" Beckett said, mostly because he couldn't remember that man's actual name. He could recite pretty much every bone and major vessel in the human body, but names continued to escape him.

"Dr. Campbell, is that you?"

"Yeah, it's me. I think my TA brought you some organs yesterday—a heart and a liver? They were… uhh… misplaced or misdirected or something."

"Yeah, I have them here. Based on the extent of tissue degeneration, both have been out of the body for at least 30 hours, which means that the heart is no longer viable. The liver, however, is still good for a day or two. You know, the strange thing is, organs are heavily coded because they go bad so quickly and when you have a donor, UNOS—"

"Yeah, okay, whatever. I've got another heart for you, but I'm thinking that it'll only be good for a few more hours. What about the liver? Any way you can extend the viability?"

"Wait—*another* heart? Where did it come from? How long ago was it removed?"

Beckett shook his head and closed his eyes.

"No idea. I'm thinking with this new hospital wing, things got all fucked-up—I'm still looking into it. What about the liver? Can you stretch it out?"

"Yeah, we can perfuse it with a combination of antifreeze and glucose—"

"Okay, Lab Guy, do what you can. And the heart is on my desk, see if you can't send one of your minions to pick it up."

Beckett didn't wait for a reply; he hung up the phone and then quickly left his office.

***

The Lab Guy was right, of course. It was next to impossible for an organ to show up unintentionally on his desk. It wasn't as if a low-level EMS guy just read the address wrong; all organs for transplant were registered through the United Network for Organ Sharing—UNOS—long before they were removed from the donor. These were… not from there.

And he knew that if he could figure out where they'd come from, he'd be that much closer to determining who had sent them.

This was Beckett's third time visiting the McEwing Transplant Unit, which, in his estimation, was three times too many. And when he pressed the intercom button beside the door, he felt as if he were on a first name basis with the secretary who replied.

Only Beckett had a problem with names; the few that he could remember included his own and the ones that were represented by the tattoos on his ribs.

"Hi, I was here yesterday looking for Dr... uh... Singh? I have a couple of follow-up questions for him. My name's Dr. Campbell, by the way."

There was a pause that went on too long for Beckett's liking.

"I'm sorry, Dr. Campbell, but the director isn't in right now. But I can relay a message if you want?"

Beckett looked around to make sure that no one was within hearing distance and then leaned close to the microphone.

"Tell him that I've got another organ—I'll wait."

"Unfortunately, Dr. Campbell, as I said, the director's not in right now so you'll have to—"

"Tell him that if he doesn't want to talk to me about these organs, I'm sure someone at *The Times* will. It'll make a nice follow-up to the piece they did on the ribbon-cutting ceremony just the other day. And, considering that I'm on the board of directors of this Goddamn place, maybe he should take what I have to say seriously. What do you think, Sally?"

Another pause, but instead of the woman coming back on the intercom, Beckett heard a buzz.

He frowned and pushed the door open.

Chapter 15

"I DON'T LIKE BEING threatened, Dr. Campbell," Dr. Singh said as he and Beckett strode down the empty hallway.

"And I don't like having organs dumped on my desk," Beckett replied. The man stopped suddenly and turned to face Beckett.

He had pale blue eyes that stood out on his dark skin; eyes that presently bored into Beckett.

"What's your game here, Dr. Campbell? You want money? Funding? Because let me tell you, the McEwing Foundation didn't even give us enough to open on time. You think that we wanted to do the grand opening and then close the doors immediately afterward? You think that was the plan? You think I wanted to make up some bullshit story for the press so that they wouldn't be all over us?"

Beckett blinked several times and wished at that moment that he'd actually paid attention at the board of directors meeting rather than picking fluff from his navel.

Still…

"What the fuck is wrong with you?" he asked.

When the director just gawked, Beckett was forced to bite his tongue. He wanted to tell this guy off; Dr. Singh was worried about funding and how the press perceived things when Beckett had just told him that he had two hearts that were suitable for donation that had been ruined and a liver that was destined to end up in the incinerator.

But he didn't.

Beckett might be short-tempered, but he also recognized when being civil was more likely to get him what he wanted, no matter how it pained him to act out of character.

And given the stakes, he saw little choice in the matter.

"Look, man, all I want to do was find out why these organs are getting sent to my office—that's it. I want to know where they come from, so UPS or FedEx or whoever the hell dropped them off can get them to where they need to go. So people don't *die*."

Now it was the director's turn to shake his head.

"Well, Dr. Campbell, like I told you, I don't know—"

This is going nowhere...

He hated when doctors played politicians and vice-versa.

Beckett suddenly held up the white vinyl bag with 'ORGAN DONOR FOR TRANSPLANT' written on the side.

"Have you seen this before?"

Dr. Singh stared at it for a moment.

"Yeah, that looks like the type of bags we have... they came with some of the other equipment we purchased—thrown in as part of the package. You know how these medical device companies work: buy ten dialysis machines at thirty K apiece, and they'll throw in some swag."

Beckett raised an eyebrow.

"And are you missing any? Two, to be precise?"

The director sighed and his shoulders slumped. For the first time since they'd met, the man seemed to let his guard down. And as he did, his perfect hair and skin melted away, leaving behind just a man in his mid-sixties who was clearly exhausted of playing dual roles.

Beckett had seen this before.

He'd known doctors who spent considerable effort trying to be something that other people wanted them to be—a physician by day, and someone who was smiling all the time and receptive to donors by night—when all they wanted to do was relax in sweatpants and drink a cold Budweiser.

In the end, it had torn them apart, leading to severe depression and extended leaves of absence.

Yeah, Beckett knew the feeling and he had to fight the sudden urge to rub the tattoos under his right arm.

"To be honest, I have no idea. I doubt even our storage room staff have any clue as to how many bags are supposed to be in there. It's just been such a shit show ever since we started having these funding problems."

Now that the real Dr. Singh had come out, Beckett started to take pity on the man.

"I understand, Dr. Singh—trust me, I do. I hate all this bureaucratic bullshit as much as the next guy. But do you think I could take a look? I mean, I'm not out to get anybody here, I'm just trying to make sure that no other perfectly good organs are wasted."

The director looked around before turning back to Beckett.

"I'll tell you what; if you want, you can go down the hall and look in the storage room yourself. Like I said, though, it's a fucking shit show in there and I doubt you'll find anything. But if you're looking for more of those bags that's where they *should* be. Other than that, the only thing I can suggest is to reach out to UNOS. See if they can help."

As he spoke, the man's shoulders started to stiffen and he regained his previous composure, posture, and identity.

"Thanks," Beckett said, and then he reached out and slapped the man on the back.

The director frowned, nodded, and then started down the hall in the opposite direction.

"I have a meeting to get to, so please see yourself out when you're done."

With that, Dr. Singh bowed his head and left Beckett to his thoughts.

Chapter 16

THE DIRECTOR WASN'T LYING; if anything, he was understating the shit show that was the storage locker.

The twenty by twenty-foot room was located at the very end of a long, nondescript hallway. It was labeled as a Supply Room, but after opening the door, Beckett quickly realized that it would be more appropriately defined as a junk room. It reminded him of the drawer that everyone had in their kitchen, the one filled with crap that you never needed, but for some reason was hesitant to throw out: elastics, chopsticks, staples without a matching stapler, and wounded paperclips.

After wading through about a metric ton of plastic tubing, Beckett found a plastic shelf at the back. Stacked on this shelf were several cardboard boxes with 'TRANSPLANT UNIT' scrawled on the side. Curious, Beckett looked for one that was already open.

He found one near the bottom against the wall. After removing it from the shelf, he sat on the floor and opened it. It took him less than 30 seconds to peel away the cellophane and realize that he was staring at a nearly full box of white vinyl cooler bags that were identical to the one that he had brought with him to the Unit.

"Well, I'll be damned."

Beckett pulled the first bag out of the box and unfolded it. Then he carefully scanned the interior. Inside, there was the ubiquitous manufacturer's tag, along with washing instructions, which he thought strange, but he also noticed a small sticker wedged in one of the seams.

Using his nails, he managed to tease it out. On the sticker, which was about the size of a postage stamp, was a seven-digit number, followed by two letters: AC.

Beckett thought about this for a moment, before concluding that it must have been some sort of inspection number.

He flipped the bag that he had brought with him inside out and, sure enough in almost the exact same location, he found a similar sticker.

A sticker with the exact same inspection number on it.

Excited now, he took another box off the shelf and tore it open. A quick search revealed that while these bags also had numbers, they finished with PT and not AC.

After snapping a few pictures, Beckett shoved the bags back in the boxes and replaced them on the shelf. Then he left the musty-smelling storage room and hurried down the hallway.

But instead of leaving as the director had suggested he should, Beckett searched around until he found the secretary's office.

She was tucked away in a room near the entrance, and when he knocked on the door, she looked up, a startled expression on her face.

That's what you get for being a dick, Beckett.

He put on his best fake smile and knocked again.

With an unwavering scowl, the woman eventually waved him in.

"How can I help you?" she snapped as soon as Beckett entered the cramped office.

"Hi there. My name is—"

"I know who you are. And my name isn't Sally, but Tracy, Tracy Allman. Is there something that I can help you with?

The director has given me strict instructions not to let anyone inside the unit until it's officially open to the public."

Beckett resisted the urge to roll his eyes. At present, it appeared that every human in the world had inexplicably lost the ability to come up with a unique sentence. All they seemed capable of was repeating the same refrains over and over again.

"No offense, but…"

"This is just my opinion…"

"Sorry to interrupt…"

Beckett cleared his throat. If charm wasn't going to get him anywhere then he had to resort to more archaic methods; mainly, bribery.

He held up a finger and with his other hand he reached into his wallet and pulled out a hundred-dollar bill.

After dramatically flattening the crumpled bill, Beckett placed it on the counter in front of Tracy Allman.

"I'm sorry for being rude earlier, it's been a long… well, week or so. I just have a simple question for you."

The woman looked at the hundred-dollar bill on the table as if it were a rotting fish.

Whoops, Beckett thought, *maybe bribery wasn't the best approach here.*

"I'm not a hooker," she snapped.

Beckett's eyes bulged as he stared at the woman's meaty hands, the broad nose that jutted from horn-rimmed glasses.

Not sure anyone would accuse you of that, sweetheart.

"I'm sorry for being a dick, I really am. And I had no intention of overstepping, uhh, *boundaries.* But here's the thing: there are over 160,000 people waiting for organs in the US, but less than 10,000 donors. The truth is, most will die waiting to get an organ. And hearts, in particular, are exceedingly rare. Seeing as you are so good at your job, I'm sure you must have overheard mine and Dr. Singh's conversation and understand why I was so desperate to speak to him."

Something in the woman's face changed and Beckett knew that he had finally pressed the right button.

What you can't win by charm or bribery, you can acquire by guilt.

"All I want to know is who had access to the storage room over the past few days."

The woman nodded slowly.

"To be honest, it's been pretty much a ghost town around here. Aside from myself and Dr. Singh, we've had a handful of technicians setting up some equipment. That's about it."

Beckett frowned.

"No one else?"

Tracy started to shake her head, then stopped.

"Well, people from the foundation were here prior to the opening. But no other doctors or benefactors."

The McEwing *Foundation,* Beckett thought. *As in* Grant McEwing.

"Thank you," he said, taking the bill off the counter and slipping it back into his pocket. "And, Sally? Don't forget to check off 'Organ Donor' next time you renew your license."

Chapter 17

BECKETT HAD NO SOONER left the transplant unit when his cell phone started to ring. In general, he found the thing annoying—more in principle than in practice.

Who wanted to be reachable at all times during the day? Certainly not him and certainly not the residents. As a result, he usually kept a low profile, suggesting to others that his cell phone should only be called in case of an emergency.

But with everything that was happening these days, everything seemed to fit that bill.

He answered without even checking to see who was calling first.

"Beckett."

"Hey, Dr. Campbell. It's Trevor," a male voice he didn't recognize replied.

Beckett turned his gaze upward. The sun was high in the sky now, and he realized that he'd spent more time in the transplant unit than he'd thought.

"I'm not interested in taking any survey," he said flatly.

"What?"

Beckett pulled the phone away from his ear and looked at the number on the display.

"Oh, Lab Guy! Why didn't you just say that—thought you were a telemarketer."

"Yeah, *umm*, anyway, I grabbed the heart on your desk earlier and I managed to do some testing on the organs that your TA brought by yesterday."

Beckett's eyes narrowed; anything the man could tell him about who the organs belonged to might get him closer to figuring out who had sent them.

"Yeah, go ahead. I'm listening."

"Well, it's not much, but both organs belonged to a male between the ages of 18 and 30-ish. Healthy male, as far as I can tell."

Beckett chewed the inside of his lip. Organs from young people were rare, but in the case of males, there tended to be one cause of death that was more common than all others combined: car accidents.

He made a mental note to look into if there were any recent fatal car accidents in New York involving men in this age group.

"Are they from the same person?" he asked.

"Not sure; all I can say is that both are from a person or persons in the same age group. If you really want to know, I can do some genetic testing to find out."

Beckett nodded.

"I want."

"It's not gonna be cheap, Dr. Campbell."

"Can't you just run it through the general lab fund?"

"It doesn't really qualify for general lab work. Besides, I wouldn't even know how to bill the service. And something like this… something in the two- to five-thousand-dollar range will immediately be flagged."

Beckett frowned.

Five grand for a simple genetic comparison test? Shit, I can send a buccal swab to a website and get my entire DNA profile for less than a c-note.

He sighed.

"Fine. Just bill it to the pathology department, care of myself, and I'll make sure you get paid. Speaking of which, what's the status of the organs? Still viable?"

"The liver's fine—cryopreserving it—I'd say an eight out of ten. The heart is done, though."

"And you have no idea where they might have come from?"

The Lab Guy paused.

"I thought you were looking into that?"

And there's my answer.

"Shit, alright. Thanks, Lab Guy. I'll be in touch."

"Dr. Campbell, I just—"

Beckett quickly hung up the phone before Lab Guy asked him out on a date.

Five grand? Seriously?

The idea irked him. It was amazing how a private company could do something so cost-efficiently, while a publicly funded institution charged an order of magnitude more for the same task.

This line of thinking brought back something that Dr. Singh had said, about how the funding for the new transplant unit had dried up.

Beckett knew little of the McEwing Foundation other than the fact that Dr. Peter McEwing had been running the show until he'd died, and that his children were now in charge. But he recalled seeing something in the paper that Delores had shown him yesterday, not about Winston Trent, but about the McEwing Foundation.

As luck would have it, a kid with slicked hair and a soul patch was striding toward him, his face buried in a newspaper. This was something of a rare sight: a young college student reading an actual newspaper.

Beckett suspected that the kid was a vegan-environmentalist-hipster who was saving the world by using the fine print for toilet paper when he was done cursing the capitalist pigs who had written it.

As he walked by, Beckett reached out and deftly snatched the paper from the man's hands.

"Hey!" the hipster shouted.

Beckett made his eyes go wide.

"There's a… a… a vegetable fire! Quick! Go save the kumquats!" Beckett exclaimed, pointing back the way he'd come.

The man looked at him as if he were certifiably insane.

"What the fuck are you talking about? A kumquat is a fruit."

Beckett chuckled and then simply turned and started to walk away. The man moved toward him, but then changed his mind and shook his head.

"Asshole," the hipster grumbled.

"You ain't lying," Beckett shot back.

He opened the newspaper and immediately smiled.

The thing about newspapers is that when something was popular on one day, they were likely going to run the exact same thing on the next… and the day after that… and the day after that. Pretty much continually until something else of substance occurred.

And this was no exception.

The front page was dominated by Winston Trent's mugshot.

You got what you deserved…

But that wasn't what Beckett was looking for.

On the second page, he saw a black-and-white image of Sir England and Grant and Flo-Ann McEwing cutting the ribbon.

Beckett scanned the text, looking for something that the article had alluded to the day prior.

He found it in the second to last paragraph.

In addition to being the major funder for the McEwing Transplant Unit, the McEwing Foundation has also recently invested an additional two million into the New York City Renewed Life Center.

Having found the information he needed, Beckett began the monumental task of folding the paper. He gave up after a good minute of trying—it was like the world's most complex Origami swan. Eventually, he just balled it up and tossed it into the nearest trash bin.

New York City Renewed Life Center.

The place sounded like one that Sir Francis England frequented nightly to have his skin regenerated.

So, the McEwing Foundation doesn't have enough money to open the Transplant Unit on time, but they can fund the Regenerated Living Quarters or whatever the hell it's called? How does that make sense?

Sure, Beckett could look the place up, figure out exactly what the Foundation was funding. But that would require going back to his office and sitting in front of his computer.

A much better idea was to meet an old friend who was in the know and share a drink.

With a smile, Beckett took his cell phone out of his pocket and dialed a number.

"Dr. Ron? How the hell have you been?"

Chapter 18

DR. RON STRANSKY WAS already at the bar when Beckett arrived, which came as no surprise; Ron was *always* at the bar. A friend from his medical school days—Ron had been a fourth year when Beckett just started—the man liked to drink as much as he liked to have his face plastered on the cover of surgical journals.

Beckett walked over to his friend and slapped him on the back. Ron looked up at him, and Beckett did a double-take. Never accused of being one of the more attractive people in medicine—Ron had a narrow nose and thin lips, which matched his thinning hairline—what the man lacked in looks he made up for in confidence.

But even when Ron smiled at him, there was a hollowness behind his eyes. He didn't exude charisma at that moment; instead, the only thing he radiated was alcoholism.

"Dr. Campbell, what a nice surprise," Ron said, reaching out for a hug. Beckett embraced the man and cringed when he felt his ribs through the back of his shirt.

"Not much of a surprise, given that we planned to meet here for drinks," Beckett replied, his eyes drifting to the rock glass in Ron's hand. "Which I see you've already gotten a head start on. That's fine, though; you've always needed a head start to keep up with me. Also, on a related note, why the hell do you look like shit?"

Ron chuckled, which quickly degenerated into a wheeze.

"Shit, man, you look terrible," Beckett said, his voice taking on a more serious tone.

"Well, you're no Christmas Peach, either. Looks like you haven't slept in a month."

Beckett had no clue what the hell a Christmas Peach was, but Ron did have a point.

Sleep was... *eventful,* in a way it had never been before.

"Great, glad to get the niceties out of the way," Beckett said as he grabbed the barstool next to his friend. "Please tell me that you aren't drinking a shitty blended whiskey."

"You know me; I could never lie to you."

"Jack Daniels," Beckett muttered. "You know, with the money you make, you should be drinking from the top shelf."

Ron just shrugged and Beckett called the bartender over.

"A beer—anything will do."

The bartender nodded and retreated to pour his drink.

"Ah, and I can see you're still into the good stuff, as well."

"Touché."

As they waited for the bartender to return with Beckett's beer, Ron quickly addressed the elephant in the bar, which he was apt to do. Like Beckett, Ron was curt and to the point. There was no standing on ceremony between them, given how deep their friendship ran.

"So, are you finally reinstated after what happened with Craig Sloan?"

Beckett tilted his head to one side.

"Reinstated... I was never *de*-instated. But yeah, things are mostly back to normal. They're still using me sparingly as the ME, but I suspect that'll change soon. Bodies be piling up."

The bartender returned with his beer and Beckett slipped him a ten. As he drank, he stared directly at Ron.

"But that's not why I asked you here. To be blunt, Ron, I need your brain."

"Yeah, well, I do, too. You can't have it."

Beckett ignored the comment.

"You always had a knack for remembering useless knowledge… and it appears that it might finally come in handy."

"What do you want to know?"

"The McEwing Foundation… any idea where they get their money from?"

Now it was Ron's turn to raise an eyebrow, albeit one considerably thicker and bushier than Beckett's own.

"Aren't you on the board of directors for the transplant unit?"

Beckett took another gulp of beer.

"Allegedly. But I slept during most of the meetings and was hungover for the rest. Besides, I don't think where they got their money from comes up that often at those sorts of things."

Ron finished his drink and ordered another. The fact that the bartender didn't expect payment as he had for Beckett suggested that Ron already had a tab running.

Figures.

"Well, you're in luck: that is one of the few things that my addled brain can remember these days. Most of the McEwing family fortune came from their great-grandfather, John D. McEwing. He was a banker who invested in some early medical devices and treatments, mainly dialysis machines and vaccines—made a shitload of money. From there, he just continued to invest and it trickled down the line. I worked with the late Peter McEwing—he was a great doctor, just like his father. It's a shitty thing that happened to him, given that he was so young."

Beckett nodded and recalled his own interactions with Dr. McEwing. The man had been boring and awkward, but from

all accounts, he meant well. He was also an excellent doctor.
As for how he died—

"Cancer," Ron said, reading his thoughts. "Oh, I mean
officially cause of death was liver failure, but that was a
consequence of liver cancer that spread pretty much
everywhere, including his lungs and heart. It was ironic,
really, given that he needed a new liver and there were none
available to him just before they promised eight figures to the
new transplant unit. Not that he was a candidate, anyway; the
cancer would've just returned... still, a shitty way to go."

Beckett etched this factoid into his mental ledger.

"What about the other things that the foundation does? The
New York Regenerating Life Project or whatever."

Ron laughed and then wiped his mouth with the back of
his hand. He really did look terrible.

"Yeah, that was in the news a few weeks back. *The New
York City Renewed Life Center*... sounds like an old age home
but it's actually meant for youth, to help them readjust to
society."

"Readjust... you mean, like criminals?"

Ron tilted his glass and filled his cheeks with cheap
whiskey before swallowing.

"That and addicts, mostly. I mean, I don't blame them for
giving it such an obtuse name. Could you imagine trying to
get donations if they were upfront about their main delegates?
New York Halfway House for Young, Drug-Addicted Criminals. I
think you'd agree that that name doesn't have the same
appeal."

"Honesty... it's a dying breed," Beckett replied. "Cynicism,
however, apparently is alive and well. Any idea who chooses
where the money goes? Who makes the final decisions? That
sort of crap?"

Ron shrugged.

"That I don't know. But these types of foundations are usually run by a board of directors comprised of people who do nothing else but serve on *other* foundation boards— nepotism at its finest—with a sprinkling of family members thrown in."

Beckett's mind turned to Grant McEwing, the way he had been so confident in the cause of death of the submerged woman when none of the other residents even had a clue.

Things were definitely pointing at Grant as the person who had sent him the organs; after all, he had the skill set to remove them and had access to young men at the halfway house. But Beckett had stared the man in the face when he brought up the note—*Home is where the heart is*—to nothing but a blank stare.

"What's with all the questions about the foundation?" Ron asked, drawing Beckett out of his head. "You thinking about starting your own? Dr. Beckett Campbell's four-fingered guitar school for troubled youths and adolescent queers?"

Beckett laughed out loud, spraying beer on the table. He raised his missing finger and wagged it in the air.

"I'm not sure it would be much easier to get donations for a Foundation that has the words finger, youth, and adolescent queers in the name."

He chugged his beer and slapped Ron on the back.

"I should get going. I want nothing more than to get totally shit-faced on a Tuesday morning with you, but—"

"—afternoon," Ron corrected.

"Sure, afternoon… but I've got shit to do. Some of us have to work for a living—we can't all rest on our laurels."

"Rest on our laurels," Ron repeated with a snicker. "What a stupid phrase—a plant to represent victory and status. It should be a rifle or spear. Speaking of victory, what *did* happen to your finger?"

Beckett smirked at the non-sequitur.

"Hunting accident," he said, keeping with the theme. He slapped Ron on the back a second time. "Don't forget to tip the bartender and thanks for your help."

With that, Beckett started to make his way toward the door.

"Hunting accident? I thought you hated hunting."

Beckett shrugged and kept walking.

It was true that while he wasn't a fan of hunting defenseless animals, he'd recently come to realize that there was one type of hunting that he very much enjoyed.

The kind that involved bipedal prey who had already done some hunting of their own.

Chapter 19

BECKETT PUT OFF DOING any more work for the afternoon. He needed to sign off on three bodies that had arrived at the morgue earlier in the day, but none of them were urgent.

On the way home, he'd gotten a cryptic text from Suzan telling him that she had to stay late after anatomy class. She'd also asked him to wait around for her, which was odd—Suzan was independent if nothing else—but Beckett had declined.

The truth was, he just wanted to be alone for a little while. A dangerous proposition, what with his racing thoughts, but he needed time to just veg out.

He typed as much to Suzan, then shut off his phone.

Suzan would understand, or at least Beckett hoped she would. He also hoped that she'd swing by later and they'd work out their 'feelings.'

After parking in his driveway, Beckett headed up the steps to his front door.

Once inside, he inhaled deeply.

"Home sweet home," he said.

It was cheesy and cliché, but true. At home, he could be himself. At home when Suzan wasn't there, he could *really* be himself.

As he walked over to grab a beer from the fridge, he peeled off his T-shirt and tossed it on the couch. Looking down at his pasty body, and the small paunch that had started around his midsection, he thought briefly about going to the gym to work out or for a drop-in jiujitsu class.

But as soon as the golden liquid hit his lips, the thought was dashed.

He'd told Ron that he had to leave the bar to get work done, but that had been a lie. He had to leave because he didn't really feel comfortable drinking in front of him.

Ron looked like fucking death incarnate.

Beckett shuddered and took another swig of beer. As he made his way around the back of the couch and flicked on the TV, he noticed that the window above the sink was open. He made his way over and peered outside. As was common in New York, it looked out over a small alley and another brick façade.

Beckett was staring out the window, looking at the pockmarked bricks of his neighbor's domicile, when he heard a sound from behind him.

His first thought was that it was the TV, but it couldn't be; he always muted it before he went to bed in case he got up early and was inclined to watch without waking Suzan. Nothing was more annoying than ear-splitting sports highlights to wake a woman from her slumber. Besides, he'd been living in this house for almost five years and he knew every sound that it made from the creaking of the floors underfoot, to the drone of the air conditioner during hot New York summers.

And this was definitely the former. Beckett took a deep breath and glanced down at the faucet in front of him.

Thank God for Suzan's cleaning, he thought as he stared into the highly reflective material.

There, not six feet behind him, approached a figure dressed all in black.

In one smooth motion, Beckett reached out and grabbed a knife from the block and whipped around. He didn't spin in a tight circle, however, but in a wide, looping arc, which took the intruder by surprise.

Beckett instinctively grabbed the man's left wrist and twisted it behind his back before he could so much as yelp.

Then he leaned in close to the man's ear and pressed the knife point against his throbbing carotid artery.

"Who the fuck are you and what the fuck are you doing in my house?" Beckett demanded.

PART II

Surgical

Intervention

Chapter 20

"BECKETT! WHAT THE HELL are you doing?" Suzan shouted as she burst through the door.

Beckett whipped around and glared at Suzan. Her eyes darted from the kitchen knife in his hand to the scene behind him.

And then she dropped the two plastic bags of Chinese food.

"Beckett!" she shouted again as she hurried past him.

Beckett stepped in front of her, trying to block her path with his free hand. She swatted it away.

"Suzan, this fucking guy broke—"

"Get the hell out of my way," Suzan snapped. Beckett, confused now, reluctantly moved aside, but his grip on the knife didn't loosen.

What the fuck is going on here?

"This is Brent," Suzan said as she crouched.

During the entire interaction, the man in the chair, who had a shaved head and dark circles under his eyes, didn't say anything at all. There was a trickle of blood leading from one nostril to the corner of his mouth courtesy of a slap that Beckett had delivered, but ever since entering the house, he hadn't said more than two words.

"You know this man?" Beckett asked.

"This my friend, Brent Taylor," Suzan said, her own anger dissipating. Before Beckett could catch his bearings and figure out exactly what the hell was going on, Suzan ducked behind the man and started to untie the telephone cord that Beckett had used to bind him to the chair. "I told you that someone was coming by and might be staying with us for a while."

Beckett's jaw drop.

His exhausted mind was having a hard time wrapping itself around the fact that Suzan knew this man… this 'Brent Taylor.' And that she thought he could stay with them.

"What in the fuck is going on here, Suze?"

Suzan finally managed to untie the man and he rose to his feet. As Brent rubbed his wrists, which were red and raw, Beckett felt every muscle in his body tense as he prepared to pounce should this man try anything.

A friend of Suzan's or not, Beckett wasn't in the mood to get pummeled by a young punk dressed in rags.

"Why don't you sit down again," Beckett suggested. He twisted his wrist slightly as he said this, causing light to reflect off the blade in his hand.

"Put the knife away, Beckett. I told you, he's a friend. I thought maybe he could stay with us for a few days."

Beckett didn't listen, he simply looked from Suzan to Brent and back again.

"Suzan, this fucking guy broke into my house. He was fucking sneaking up on me."

Suzan glanced at Brent, who, unbelievably, still hadn't said anything.

"Are you a fucking mute? Why don't you say something? Why the hell did you break into my house?"

Brent averted his eyes and lowered his chin to his chest.

Suzan, eyes blazing, stormed over to Beckett, grabbed him by the arm, and pulled him into the kitchen. Beckett allowed himself to be led, but he didn't take his eyes off Brent for a second.

"Beckett, you tied him up? You tied Brent up and put a knife to his throat?"

Beckett finally looked away from Brent and turned to Suzan.

"What the hell, Suzan? I come home after a long day at work only to find that this asshole broke into my house. What the hell did you want me to do? Let him sneak up on me?"

"I tried texting… and calling to let you know, but your damn phone was off. Brent… he's not… he's not well, Beckett."

Beckett lifted his eyes to look at Brent again.

"No shit. What's wrong with him?"

"He… look, I knew him in high school. Back then, he was normal. But something happened… they say he fell off his bike, but his dad was a grade A asshole and I wouldn't be surprised if he had beat him up. After that," Suzan leaned in close and continued quietly, "he was different—slow. It wasn't long before people started to take advantage of him. Then, two years ago, I hear from some other friends that Brent was going to prison for dealing drugs. He didn't… someone just tricked him, Beckett. Like I said, he was a good kid. He got out yesterday, and I thought I could help him out. But I couldn't go to my mom, not with the newborn and what happened with Drake."

Beckett could barely believe what he was hearing.

"Drake? You're worried about Drake? With everything going on at the hospital, with the Internal Affairs assholes, you thought that bringing him here was a good idea? You think I need to have a fugitive in my house right now?"

Suzan shook her head.

"He's not a fugitive, Beckett. He served his time and is out on parole. I just thought he could stay with us for a while. I wanted to ask you, but..."

Beckett looked at Brent again, whose eyes were once again looked on his worn running shoes.

"Nuh-uh, there's no way," Beckett said. No matter what Brent's problems were and how close he was with Suzan, there was no change that he was letting the kid stay in his house. Not after he'd crawled through the window, not after what happened in the Virgin Gorda, not after what happened with Winston Trent, and definitely not after receiving fucking random organs on his desk with cryptic notes.

Suzan looked at him for a good ten seconds before answering.

"Seriously? Beckett, he needs help."

"Damn right it does. But I'm not the man to help him. I'm sorry, Suzan but he can't stay here." A thought suddenly occurred to him. "But there is somewhere he *can* stay. There is this place, the... *uhh*... New York Revitalized Life thingy that helps people like him get back on their feet. It's not too far from here, and I know I can get him a spot."

Suzan's jaw dropped.

"A fucking halfway house? Let me get this straight: you want him to go to a place full of ex-cons who are just going to manipulate him again? Get him arrested and thrown back in jail? Is that what you're proposing?"

Beckett felt his anger rising.

"I'm trying to help him, Suzan, but like I said, he's not staying here."

Suzan pressed her lips together tightly and then walked over to Brent and hooked an arm through his.

"Well if he's going, then I'm going with him. Because if he can't stay, then neither will I."

Beckett looked at Suzan's face for any indication that she might be bluffing.

She wasn't.

But Beckett was in no mood to negotiate.

"Fine. Go with him—just don't be late for class tomorrow."

The barb was intentional; Suzan hated when he treated her like his TA and not his girlfriend.

She led Brent to the door and opened it. Then she looked back, clearly giving Beckett an opportunity to change his mind, before slamming it closed behind them.

"Fuck!" Beckett swore. "What the fuck just happened?"

Chapter 21

BECKETT HOVERED OVER THE bodies, a gleaming scalpel in his hand. He was wearing his blue smock and a white mask that covered his nose and mouth. Both were speckled with blood. He moved to the first corpse, a man in his late-30s whose body was in relatively good shape.

His head wasn't.

The mans' skull was collapsed inward and his face squished as if made of Play-Doh. But Beckett wasn't concerned with any of this.

He used the scalpel and performed a quick Y incision and then, with hands buried in thick, black rubber gloves, he pulled the skin of the man's chest apart. Then he grabbed the Sawzall from the table beside him and began cutting away at the man's ribcage. The room was suddenly filled with the sound of a whirring blade coupled with a high-pitched whine as Beckett cut through the ribs adjacent to the sternum.

With a grunt, Beckett grabbed both sides of the ribcage and cracked them open like a turkey wishbone.

After switching out the Sawzall for his trusty scalpel, he set about cutting first through the thoracic cavity and then the pericardial cavity. Once the heart was exposed, he carefully severed the aorta, the pulmonary artery, and the superior vena cava. After gliding the blade behind the heart to sever all remaining connective tissue, Beckett reached inside the body and removed the man's heart.

Inexplicably, it was still warm in his gloved hand.

Beckett placed the heart in a plastic biohazard bag and then nestled the package on the dry ice that nearly filled the organ transplant cooler.

Satisfied, he moved on to the next cadaver, that of Donnie DiMarco. Unlike Craig Sloan, this man's face was intact, but he had the characteristic features of a man who'd drowned: sunken eyes, blue lips, pale flesh.

Beckett repeated the process with this man, but instead of just removing his heart, he removed the man's liver, as well.

The next cadaver belonged to Ray Reynolds and, lying beside him was, the white hulk: Bob Bumacher.

He removed both of their hearts before moving on to the final two bodies: Boris Brackovich, whose neck was a tattered mess, and finally, Winston Trent, whose only sign of the torture he'd endured were small cuts on his wrists.

He removed their hearts and livers and placed them in the organ transplant cooler.

When he was done, Beckett sighed and wiped the sweat from his brow as he observed his handiwork.

Six bad men who had done bad things and would've continued to do bad things if Beckett hadn't intervened.

Sometimes even a doctor had to take a life to save a life.

Or six.

Beckett was about to lay down the scalpel when he heard a sound from behind him and whipped around.

It was Suzan and she was staring at him, her eyes wide.

"What have you done? Beckett, what in the world of you done?"

Chapter 22

BECKETT AWOKE DRENCHED IN sweat. There was a weight pushing down on his chest, and he could barely breathe.

He half-expected it to be Brent Taylor sitting on top of him and he looked to his left for Suzan for help.

But neither was in the room with him; he was alone.

With a gasp, Beckett managed to fully inflate his lungs. And with this, snippets of his dream came flooding back. They were incomplete, just flashes of blood, of a scalpel blade, of a bone saw, but they were enough.

Beckett raised his right arm and ran the fingers of his left hand across the tattoos that marked his ribs.

As he did, he muttered the names of those he'd taken.

"Craig Sloan… Donnie DiMarco… Ray Reynolds… Bob Bumacher… Boris Brackovich… Winston Trent…"

He did this several times until his breathing returned to normal.

Only then did he check the clock and was surprised to see that it was nearly six in the morning.

Despite the horrible nightmare, he had managed to sleep the whole night through, which was something of an anomaly with him. Beckett peeled the sweaty sheet off his body and then rose. With a grunt, he slowly made his way to the bathroom and stared at himself in the mirror.

This was becoming a habit of his, a sort of tangible introspection that was relatively new. Evidently, taking the lives of six people—despicable, murderous creatures— changed you in more ways than one.

Beckett was taken aback by his own reflection. It wasn't his matted hair, or his pale cheeks, or even the dark circles beneath his eyes that gave him pause; it was his eyes, themselves. Normally a vibrant blue, they appeared paler than usual.

Paler, and more empty.

"You're just being melodramatic," he muttered under his breath.

I know what you are… I know what you did…

For some reason, when the words from the yellow pieces of paper echoed in his head, they did so in Suzan's voice.

Beckett showered quickly and then prepared himself a pot of coffee. After pushing the Brent Taylor debacle from his mind, he thought about what he'd uncovered yesterday, that the bags were from the McEwing Transplant Unit and that the organs belonged to a young male.

It wasn't much to go on, but it was something. And even as a child, Beckett had been good at solving puzzles. Usually, however, the stakes weren't this high.

***

"Morning, Delores," Beckett said as he passed her desk.

The woman glanced up as he approached, a look of surprise on her face.

"A little early for you, isn't it, Dr. Campbell?"

She wasn't wrong about that. Typically a late riser, lately, given his fitful sleep, Beckett had had the urge to get out of his house as soon as he could.

"What can I say, damn bedbugs can me up all night," he said, but there was no humor in his voice.

Regardless, Delores smiled.

"Hey, did you see Suzan here earlier? I've got a class in about a half hour, and I was hoping she'd be able to fill in for me so that I can catch up on my beauty sleep."

Delores shook her head.

"Sorry, Dr. Campbell. I only got in twenty minutes ago and you're the first person I've seen. Besides Dr. Hollenbeck, of course."

Beckett nodded. Dr. Hollenbeck, the director of the pathology department, was 300 years old if he was a day, borderline senile, and spent every waking moment in the hospital.

Maybe he *put the organs on my desk. Maybe Dr. Hollenbeck is moonlighting as a white coat in the organ transplant unit,* Beckett thought. *And maybe, just maybe, he got confused and removed a heart when he was supposed to take out the spleen and mistook my office as the lab.*

It was improbable, but not impossible: the man had cataracts as thick as manhole covers.

"Thanks," Beckett grumbled, shaking his head. "If you see Suzan, please tell her to come to my office."

With that, Beckett hurried to his office at the end of the hallway. It only registered later that he didn't have to unlock the door.

Briefcase in hand, he stepped into the room and then froze.

There, sitting on his desk, was a plain cardboard box.

Beckett's heart started thumping in triple time and he felt as if his diaphragm had been attached to a live wire.

Please don't be another one, please don't be another one, please don't be another one…

But when Beckett made his way around to the front of his desk, he knew that whatever deity presided over him had failed to answer his pleas.

His racing heart fell into the pit of his stomach.

"Fuck," he whispered, staring at his name typed on the top of the box.

And then he yelled the word. Before storming out of the office and heading back to Delores, he threw his bag onto the chair so hard that it nearly toppled.

His blood was boiling now and even though Beckett knew that he was on the verge of losing control, he was helpless to prevent it.

Somebody was fucking with him, toying with him, playing a sadistic game with the lives of others.

Somebody who knew what he'd done, who knew what he was.

"Delores!" he screamed. "Delores! Who the fuck was in my office?"

Chapter 23

"I… I… I DON'T know," Delores stammered. She looked frightened, an expression that Beckett hadn't seen on her jovial face before.

And yet, he couldn't stem his rage.

"Someone was in my office," he barked. "And I want to know who it was."

Delores just stared at him, her eyes blinking, her mouth opening and closing like a guppy, but she said nothing.

"Are there cameras in my office?"

When Delores just blinked again, Beckett leaned over her desk.

"I asked if there were cameras in my office?"

"No, I don't… I don't think so," the secretary managed at last.

Beckett ground his teeth in frustration and turned his eyes skyward. He searched the drop ceiling for a camera and eventually saw a small dark globe in the entrance of the hallway.

"There," Beckett snapped. "Right there. That's a fucking camera."

More blinking eyes and puckered lips.

"Can you call somebody? Can you call somebody and get me footage from that camera?"

"I don't know if I—"

"*Just fucking call someone!*" Beckett screamed.

Delores recoiled and Beckett, still steaming, returned to his office and tore into the cardboard box. Part of him still hoped that it *wasn't* another organ, but when he saw the white vinyl bag…

"Goddamnit," he said as he opened the bag. Inside was another heart.

Three hearts, three dead people.

Beckett tried to swallow, but his throat was suddenly too dry.

Victims — three hearts, three victims.

He shook the thought away. There was no proof that these were victims... *yet.*

Beckett found the corresponding yellow note stuck between the cardboard box and the cooler and pulled it out.

Wherever you go, go with all your heart, it read.

Frustrated by the nonsensical saying, Beckett balled it up and tossed it into the trash.

He didn't even bother looking for a hidden message this time.

Where are these goddamn organs coming from?

Beckett's eyes rested on the pale pink heart in the clear biohazard bag as he contemplated what to do next.

Calling the cops and reporting the organs was out of the question — whether these hearts were taken from the scrap heap or from living people, whoever was sending them knew too much about Beckett.

He debated calling the lab guy again, but the last time they'd spoken, the man had sounded suspicious — and rightfully so.

His thoughts suddenly returned to the most common reason why the transplant unit received organs from young people in the first place.

Maybe I can *call the cops, but not to tell them about the organs,* Beckett thought. *Maybe I can just ask them a question.*

Beckett pulled his cell phone out of his pocket, knowing that no matter how discrete he was going to be, the call would likely come back to haunt him. Especially given his connection to Damien Drake and the problems the man was now facing.

But he was running out of options. The longer it took to figure out where these organs were coming from and who was sending them, the higher the body count.

There was one person in the NYPD, however, someone he'd worked with in the past that he thought he could still trust.

Beckett scrolled through his contacts until he came across the name he was looking for. After a brief hesitation, he clicked dial.

The phone rang several times before a male voice answered.

"Detective Dunbar."

"Dunbar, it's Beckett… Beckett Campbell," he replied hesitantly.

"Beckett! How are you? How was your vacation?"

Beckett closed his eyes and an image of Donnie DiMarco's body floating below the surface of the water, his eyes wide, his mouth slack, filled his mind.

"It was… *eventful*. How're you doing?"

Dunbar paused and when he spoke again his tone had become less enthusiastic.

"Ehhh, okay, I guess. Stressed, dealing with this Drake shit. It's been—well, I guess you know how it's been, given that he's your friend. I'm just… I'm just exhausted."

In truth, Beckett didn't know how *it* was. In fact, after what had gone down with Ray Reynolds and the Church of Liberation, mainly Beckett losing his finger and nearly dying from ethanol poisoning, he'd tried to distance himself from Drake. But he'd been drawn back to deal with Bob Bumacher and Boris Brackovich, both of whom were involved in a human trafficking and sex slave ring.

He loved Drake like a brother, but given his newest... *hobby*... Beckett had to sever ties with the man; bad luck and bad news followed him around like the plague. Drake was like the King Midas of scatology; instead of turning everything into gold, everything he touched turned to shit.

"But enough about me," Dunbar continued, "What's up, Beckett?"

Beckett chewed the inside of his lip and chose his words carefully.

"As you've probably heard, the new McEwing Transplant Unit just recently opened and I'm on the board of directors. We were discussing the discrepancy between our records of young people who chose to be organ donors, the rate of car accidents, and the number of organs we actually receive. I'm wondering if their stickers aren't accidentally peeling off their driver's licenses."

Beckett cringed; it was a horrible, circuitous way of getting around to what he really wanted to know. And it was pretty fucking stupid, too.

"Well, *uhh*, not sure if I can help you there—I'm a homicide detective, Beckett."

"Yeah, I know, it's just... I'm just grasping at straws here, Dunbar. I'd like to see one of the licenses from a young person who died in a car accident just to make sure. Do you know of any car accidents that happened lately, specifically those involving males between the ages of 18 and 35?"

Beckett closed his eyes and shook his head.

Specifically... you moron.

"Uhh, I can check if you want. Make a call or two. That it? That why you rang?"

"That's it. I know this is a strange request, but I wasn't sure who to reach out to, given my connection with Drake and his current… *issues*. Oh, and if you have any skin tags or unsightly rashes you want me to examine, I'm your guy. Free pathology for you and your crew!"

Dunbar chuckled and Beckett breathed a sigh of relief.

"All right, if I discover any plantar warts, I'll come see you. Take care, Beckett. I'll be in touch."

"Yeah, you too."

Beckett stared at his phone for a moment after the call had ended before putting it in his pocket.

Then he rubbed his eyes and looked at the schedule that Suzan had taped to his desk.

Class was starting in ten minutes, and while it was probably the last place Beckett wanted to be right now, there was one person he needed to see.

He had several specific questions for one of the new residents, one whose name just happened to match that of the new transplant unit.

Chapter 24

ON HIS WAY TO class, Beckett called Suzan twice, leaving a message the second time. His tone had come off as apologetic, he knew, but he didn't go as far as to actually apologize.

After all, slow or not, Brent Taylor *had* broken into his house and sneaked up on him. The young man was lucky that all he'd received was a bloody nose.

Others had received far worse.

Even though Suzan hadn't answered either of his calls, Beckett was still disappointed to find that she wasn't in the classroom with the residents when he entered.

"Morning," he grumbled. Several of the residents replied with a good morning of their own, but Beckett ignored them.

He was only here for one reason and one reason only: Grant McEwing. Everything else he was about to do and say was part of a charade.

If Grant was the one sending him the organs, playing this sadistic game, then Beckett would play along, for the time being.

But by the time it was all over, he'd be the one who was calling the shots.

With a broad smile, he held up a stack of papers.

"Test time!" he exclaimed.

Almost immediately, the smiles fell off the residents' faces and hands shot into the air.

"Put your hands down, this isn't the Third Reich. Besides, I already know what you're going to say: *oh*, Dr. Campbell, yesterday you told us that this residency was different, that there weren't gonna be any tests, blah, blah, blah. But here's the thing: while I don't believe in this shit, the department, and the department head, Dr. Hollenbeck, are stuck in the Jurassic Era. So, this here," he shook the stack of pages in his hand, "is the R-1 final theory exam. And you're going to take it today."

This was new grounds, even for him. While it was true that he loathed the traditional testing structure, the department decreed that all residents needed to pass the final theory and practical exams to move on to year two.

Still, there was nothing stating that Beckett couldn't *help* them along their way.

Well, actually, there was. Beckett just chose to ignore this fact as he did with most of the bureaucratic and archaic nonsense that was part and parcel with an educational institution.

"Final?" one of the two women in the class, Maria, or Mary, or something like that gasped. "How can we take the final? We haven't even studied!"

Beckett shrugged.

"It's better just to get it out of the way so you can actually learn something. Did you find yesterday interesting? Insightful? God forbid, did you actually learn something of value?"

Several residents nodded, a gesture that Beckett mimicked.

"All right then, I see that we've got a couple chicken hawks in the room. Well, yesterday was just a taste of what classes are going to be like this year. And, if you were paying attention, you should be able to answer each and every one of the very basic, and very boring, questions on the exam."

Margo started to protest again, but Beckett shook his head.

"If you don't like it, go see Dr. Hollenbeck, bring him some prune juice and Metamucil. Problem is, I've got tenure so there's not much he can do about it. What he'll most likely do is transfer you to—God forbid—one of the other forensic pathology instructors." Beckett shuddered. "So just write the damn test—*please*. Trust me, I'm sure you'll all do fine. In fact, I *assure* you."

With that, he handed out the tests and then took a seat at his desk. After confirming that all the residents were begrudgingly starting to scribble away at the sheets of paper in front of them, Beckett flicked on his computer.

He was surprised to find an email from the lab guy waiting.

Beckett didn't like emails. He didn't like texts either; he preferred phone calls. You can trace an email, there was a record of a text, but phone calls... there's no way to tell what actually took place during the call.

Thankfully, this email is simple enough.

I can confirm that the first liver and heart came from the same individual. Also, someone came by to retrieve the liver. Someone from the transplant unit—said they found a match.

The cheeky bastard even signed off as the Lab Guy.

Someone came to get the liver? Dr. Singh, maybe? Or that salad-finger guy Sir England?

Beckett debated writing back to clarify but then decided against it. No paper trail for this one.

Instead, he rose to his feet and made his way into the hallway. He was aware that the residents were staring at him, but he didn't care. He didn't give a shit if they cheated on their tests, not that he thought they would. He was more concerned with their problem-solving skills than with their ability to regurgitate useless factoids that one could look up on the internet in seconds.

Once in the hallway, he pulled his cell phone out and started to dial the Lab Guy's number.

He wanted to know who had picked up the organ and how a match could have possibly been made given that it wasn't in the UNOS system or any other, for that matter.

But Beckett hesitated. Calling and asking would only make the Lab Guy even more suspicious. Perhaps suspicious enough to start asking questions of his own...

His thoughts turned to the secretary at the transplant unit, the one who'd scorned him for trying to bribe her.

I can ask him in person, maybe offer him a little cookie to keep his mouth shut.

Just as Beckett slipped the phone back into his pocket, he caught sight of someone approaching in his periphery.

Suzan.

Beckett's first instinct was to make a joke, to make light of the situation as he often did, but he decided against the idea. Something told him that if he made a joke now, he would likely find himself missing more than just part of his finger by day's end.

A similarly-shaped appendage, perhaps, but not a finger.

"Suzan, I'm sorry. I was just—"

"Save it," she spat. "Brent's gone."

"What? What do you mean, *gone*?"

Suzan's scowl deepened.

"Last night, I checked him into the halfway house you suggested, but when I went this morning to take him out to breakfast, he was gone—and nobody would tell me where he went."

Chapter 25

"THAT'S IT, PUT YOUR pencils down," Beckett said as he entered the classroom, this time with Suzan in tow.

Several of the residents looked up at him as if you were joking, but Beckett quickly quashed that idea.

"I'm serious. Test's over."

Beckett scanned their faces, waiting, wanting one of them to say that they still had more time. Thankfully, no one did—not even Margaret. This was unexpected, but what was more surprising was Grant McEwing. The man was sitting comfortably in his chair, the test booklet closed in front of him, his fingers interlaced on top.

"Suzan is going to come by and collect the tests—that's it for today. I know, I know; yesterday you chopped up bodies for a few hours and today you wrote your final exam. I assure you, the workload will increase over time; we're starting slow, but things will build. And while my methods may be unconventional, almost all of my residents have gone on to hold prestigious positions—several of which as department heads straight out of residency—across the country. So, stick with me and you'll be rewarded."

At this point, despite his speech, Beckett was almost positive that at least one of them would complain to Dr. Hollenbeck, but he didn't give a shit.

After all, he had tenure and the senile bastard was just as likely to forget about the complaint the moment the resident left the room as he was to act on it.

And, besides, Beckett had more important things to think about now.

Like, figure out where the goddamn organs were coming from and what happened to Brent Taylor. Sure, the man had broken into his house, but he *was* Suzan's friend. And if she was this torn up about him, then it was Beckett's duty to help her out... wasn't it?

He exhaled loudly, which drew the attention of a male resident as he walked passed.

"Dr. Campbell?" the man with hawkish features asked in a tentative voice. Beckett waited for him to continue and eventually he did. "Can I ask you something?"

Beckett's reply was immediate.

"No."

"But I just—"

"I said, no. Now's not a good time."

Suzan, who was in the process of stacking the tests, shot him a look and Beckett immediately regretted his reply.

Sure, his methods were unconventional, but Beckett always had the residents' best interests at heart. And while he liked to rib them, tease them, his actions weren't cruel, they served a purpose: mainly, to challenge them and their assumptions in order to generate a better, more capable forensic pathologist.

But recently... he'd just been mean.

Beckett opened his mouth to call the man back, but he had already left the room.

"What's wrong with you?" Suzan asked now that they were alone. Beckett lowered his eyes to the missing digit on his right hand and he rubbed the numb flesh absently. "Ever since... ever since the Virgin Gorda, you've been acting differently. This isn't like you, Beckett. I mean, no one would ever accuse you of being the most compassionate or empathetic guy in the room, but you turned Brent away yesterday without even a discussion. I wouldn't have brought him to you if I thought you were going to do that."

Beckett sighed and rubbed his eyes. He didn't feel great about what had transpired with Brent, despite the man breaking into his house, but there were more pressing things on his mind.

"There was another delivery," he said, without looking up. "Another heart."

Suzan recoiled.

"What? Beckett... you have to tell someone. There's something... this isn't right."

Beckett's eyes shot up.

"I did—I told *you*."

Suzan threw up her hands.

"The police, Beckett; you need to call the police. Can't you be serious, just for once?"

"I *am* serious, Suzan. And I can't call the police—you *know* why. I bet it's one of those assholes that are gunning for my job who are sending the organs. They're just waiting for me to go to the cops, to alert Internal Affairs. This time, IA won't just 'suggest' that I go for a vacation, but they'll make it permanent. They might even reopen the whole Craig Sloan thing. I'm just going to have to figure this out by myself."

By myself... the words of an unintentional, but they stung Suzan just the same.

"Yourself, huh? So, what am I, then? Just a TA? Just a fucking hired hand?"

She was more than that to Beckett—*much* more. But Beckett couldn't get it out of his head that if he was going to go down for the things he'd done, that she would go down with him. It was more than that, too; every time she saw his tattoos, he felt guilty. Not so much for the men's lives he'd taken, but as a reminder that he was lying to her.

That he couldn't be himself around her—his *true* self. And one thing Beckett prided above nearly everything else, was being honest.

"I guess so," he said. And then he shoved the tests in her direction. "See if you can get these marked by the end of the day."

The hurt on Suzan's face was almost more than he could handle, and it was all he could do to hold his ground. It was time to start distancing himself from her, Beckett knew.

Suzan opened her mouth and looked as if she were about to say something, but then her jaw snapped closed. She grabbed the tests, tucked them under her arm and left.

"Fuck," Beckett groaned when he was finally alone. The last thing he wanted to do was hurt Suzan, but a little hurt now was better than a lot of hurt later.

With a heavy exhale, he rose to his feet and was about to make his way to the door when his phone started to ring.

"What?"

"Beckett? It's Dunbar. I looked into the car accidents like you asked."

Beckett sat back down.

"Sorry, just been a long day already. What'd you find out, Dunbar?"

"So, *uhh*, it's strange but there've been no fatal accidents involving young people over the past week or so. There was an old guy who had a stroke while driving and veered into a tree. Pronounced brain dead at the scene by one of your guys. His wallet was still in evidence, and I took a peek—he was an organ donor, and the sticker was, *uhh*, stuck pretty good. Not sure if that helps."

Beckett felt his heart sink.

Even though he knew from the get-go that it was unlikely the organs were from cadavers—*I know what you are, I know what you did*—this pretty much sealed it.

"Yeah, it helps, Dunbar," Beckett replied. "Thanks. I was just grasping at straws, anyway. Take care."

Dunbar started to say something, but Beckett had already hung up the phone.

Suzan was right, of course; he *had* to tell somebody—either that, or he had to *do* something about it.

People were being killed; *young* people.

Beckett opted for the latter.

Chapter 26

"Ron? It's Beckett."

"Two times in as many days? Either you've got a crush on me or you need a favor."

"Well, my type isn't usually sickly looking men with drinking problems. But, you know me, I'm always looking for a new experience," Beckett said. He didn't feel in the mood to joke around but knew that this was part of the game.

A major reason that Ron was so fond of Beckett, he'd realized long ago, was that the man lived vicariously through him. It wasn't just the lifestyle, but also Beckett's ability to say whatever he wanted to whomever he wanted. This was one of the mitigating factors in pushing Beckett into a discipline that didn't require interaction with patients. Ron, on the other hand, had a front facing profession, one that forced him to constantly put on a face.

Which was why he drowned himself in drink, Beckett also concluded. Keeping two different personas was an exhausting task.

"And as *you* know, I'm in a steady relationship with my friend Jack… Jack Daniels. What can I do for you, Beckett?"

"You still have your connections at UNOS?"

"Yeah, the two head honchos over there owe me a favor. Those assholes tried to slip a liver riddled with metastases into a 14-year-old kid. What's up?"

"Just wondering if you can do a little digging for me… see if you can find out if a stray liver has popped up over the past few days. Under the radar, of course."

Ron cleared his throat before replying.

"Popped up, hmm? Sure, I'll ask around."

"Thanks, Ron. I owe you a drink… or six."

***

The Lab Guy met Beckett outside the main lab building. Dressed in a white lab coat, the man's appearance reaffirmed his moniker: he had thick glasses and greasy hair tucked behind his ears.

He also had a minor stutter, Beckett noticed, that seemed more prominent in person than it did over the phone.

"D-Dr. Campbell?"

Beckett skipped the niceties; he'd played that game with Ron and didn't feel like stepping up to the plate again so soon.

"Who picked up the liver?" Beckett asked as he followed the man into the lab. He made sure that the door was closed behind them and that they were alone before continuing. "Who was it?"

Lab Guy shrugged.

"No clue. He was in and out in just a minute. Said he knew you, said that it was okay. Should I—"

Beckett shook his head. He already had Ron on the case.

"Naw, it's fine. Don't worry about it."

"But why—"

Beckett shook his head again, more deliberately this time.

"Above your pay grade."

"Everything's above my pay grade," Lab Guy muttered.

Beckett placed a hand on the man's shoulder.

"Speaking of which, I've got a couple of other things I need you to do for me. With discretion, of course."

Lab Guy's face contorted.

"I'm not sure—"

"I have no problem writing a letter of recommendation, in case another position—say, head of lab stuff—comes up. You might have heard some rumors about me, but one thing is certain: I still hold some clout here."

Lab Guy looked as if he was about to say something, but then he closed his mouth and nodded.

"What do you need me to do?" he said with a sigh.

"Incinerate the heart. Pretend you never saw it."

"What? Why?"

"Above your pay grade," Beckett repeated, placing the organ donor cooler that he'd brought with him on the table. "I want you to run some genetic tests on the two other hearts and then get rid of them, as well."

Lab Guy's eyes bulged so dramatically that Beckett could practically hear them squish up against his thick spectacles.

"Are you—wait, do you—"

"Above—"

"—my pay grade," Lab Guy finished for him.

Beckett clapped him on the back and smiled.

"And who says that an old dog can't learn new tricks."

Chapter 27

BECKETT RETURNED TO HIS office after meeting with Lab Guy, but as he approached he felt a knot twist in his stomach.

Delores was sitting at her desk, her head down as she used the first finger of each hand to peck away at her keyboard. He'd known the woman for the better part of four years now—unlike many of the other doctors, he opted not to have a personal secretary—and they'd always had a pleasant, albeit superficial relationship.

Until he'd blown up at her for something that was in no way her fault, that is. And it most definitely *wasn't* her fault; she wasn't, after all, a gatekeeper. People were free to walk the halls as much as they liked, and the fact that she hadn't seen who had delivered the organs was not her purview.

It was also very much unlike him to explode at all; Beckett dealt with stress mainly by cracking jokes and teasing others. But ever since the Virgin Gorda…

"Dr. Campbell?" Delores said, poking her head up from her computer. Beckett raised his eyes and was dismayed to see that there was actual fear in the woman's pale face. "I found —
"

Beckett stopped the woman by raising a finger.

"Delores, who's your favorite actor?"

The woman squinted at him.

"Excuse me?"

"Who is your favorite actor?" Beckett repeated.

"I… I dunno… maybe Tom Hardy?"

Beckett grimaced.

"Okay, who's your favorite B level actor, then?"

Delores paused again. She was clearly confused by this line of questioning but was averse to upsetting Beckett again.

"Chris Hemsworth?"

Beckett questioned whether or not Chris Hemsworth was a B actor—he was an A minus at worst—but it was still something he thought he might be able to swing.

He parked this information in his brain and then changed the subject.

"Good choice. Now, what were you going to tell me?"

The confusion slid off Delores's face and she became serious again.

"You know that video you asked for? The security footage? I called in a favor with the older gentleman at the security desk and managed to get a copy. It should be in your email."

Beckett felt his heart rate quicken. It appeared as if he might get to the end of this morbid mystery sooner rather than later.

And, if he was being perfectly honest with himself, a tiny part of him was disappointed; Beckett had hoped for a greater challenge.

The majority of his being, including his now tingling fingertips, however, was undeniably excited. It had been three days since he'd put an end to the sick bastard that was Wilson Trent and he could feel the urge to kill returning.

He felt like a 2L bottle of Pepsi that was slowly being shaken and the pressure from the CO_2 was about to reach a head.

"Thanks," Beckett said putting his arm on top of Delores's hand for a brief moment before pulling it back.

"Oh, and Dr. Campbell?"

Beckett turned back to look at her.

"Yeah?"

"A student of yours came in to speak to you? Said you were expecting him? Looks like Jay Baruchel with a shaved head?"

Beckett chuckled.

Speaking of B—and C and D—level actors...

"Grant McEwing," he said under his breath.

Delores nodded.

"Yeah, that's him. Is he... is he related to the new transplant wing?"

Beckett paused for a moment, mulling over the curious way that Delores had phrased her sentence.

How deep are Grant's ties to the Unit? Beckett wondered. *He was there for the ribbon-cutting ceremony and Ron mentioned that the Foundation usually placed family members on the Board.*

For the life of him, however, Beckett couldn't recall ever seeing him at any of the Board Meetings for the transplant unit.

"Is he related?" Beckett said at last. "Yeah, he most definitely is."

***

Beckett entered his office without even casting a glance in Grant's direction. Instead, he pretended not to notice the man and took a seat at his desk. He was eager to view the video that Delores had sent him but judged that that that wouldn't be a good idea with Grant in the room. Instead, he woke up his computer and then confirmed that the email was in his inbox. Then he reached for the stack of tests on his desks, the ones that Suzan had marked in record time, and shuffled them aimlessly.

Grant cleared his throat and Beckett finally raised his eyes. The man looked tired and his hair had started to grow in—it was patchy and matched the hair on his cheeks and chin.

"Why did you tell Delores that I was expecting you?" Beckett asked suddenly.

The corners of Grant's mouth twitched.

"I'm sorry, but I got the impression that she wouldn't let me in otherwise."

Beckett's eyes narrowed and he slowly reached for the top drawer of his desk. He opened it several inches, just wide enough for him to catch a glimpse of the scalpel in his periphery.

Grant looked very much like Jay Baruchel, at least in physical stature, and there was no question in his mind that if it came down to it, Beckett could take him.

Still, one could never be *too* careful.

"What else have you lied about, Grant?"

"What? Nothing? I just had to speak to you. I'm sorry—"

"Do you know who I am?" Beckett interjected.

Grant recoiled slightly.

"Yes, you're Dr. Campbell, the head of the forensic—"

"Do you know what I do?" Beckett snapped quickly.

Again, a minor recoil.

"I—I—"

"I asked you if you knew what I did?"

"Y-yes. You're a Senior Medical Examiner for the State of New York. You also…"

Beckett wasn't listening anymore; he was staring at the man's face, and, more specifically, his eyes. He'd looked into Donnie DiMarco's eyes moments before he slipped below the surface of the water, and he'd seen Craig Sloan's go wide before being struck by the rock.

And the others… he'd made a point of staring into their eyes before he finished them off.

Beckett was a doctor and a pragmatist. He didn't believe in the soul or afterlife, but there was something undeniably missing in all of his victims' eyes. Something that was difficult to articulate, but tangible, nonetheless.

Something dull, a flatness that he'd only witnessed a handful of times.

It was the same thing he saw in his own eyes when he stared in the mirror.

"One last thing, Grant: *wherever you go, go with all your heart*," Beckett said, focusing in on the young man's pupils.

Chapter 28

GRANT SHOOK HIS HEAD and blinked rapidly several times.

"I-I-I don't—I just came in here to—"

"To what, Grant?"

Grant suddenly sighed and his shoulders slumped. When he spoke again, he did so with his head bowed.

"I-I-I have to tell you something."

Beckett smirked and snaked a hand into the top drawer of his desk. His mind started working, trying to come up with a scenario by which he could dispatch Grant without Delores asking questions.

It doesn't have to be now, it doesn't have to be here…

Beckett's fingers were tingling so much now that he was almost trembling.

"Go ahead," he said with a grin.

Another heavy sigh.

"I have… I have this memory," Grant said. The response was so unexpected that Beckett recoiled this time.

"What?"

"I have an eidetic memory," Grant's eyes flicked at the tests still in Beckett's hand. "I wanted to tell you before you marked the tests, but I see that they're already done."

Beckett was confused as to what was going on. He'd seen *something* in the man's eyes, that much was certain, and was about to act on this when Grant had pulled a one-eighty.

An eidetic memory? What in the fuck?

"If I read something, I have perfect recall," Grant continued. "I've been accused of cheating too many times in the past… so I thought I would give you the heads-up."

"I know what an eidetic memory is. I also know that it's exceedingly rare in adults."

"Question nineteen," Grant said, looking off to one side. "What are the most common risk factors for acute aortic dissection in young people?"

Beckett didn't want to look at the test, but eventually, curiosity took over. Indeed, question nineteen was word-for-word as Grant had spoken it.

"And the answer?" Beckett asked, eyebrow raised.

"Marfan syndrome, bicuspid aortic valves, and larger aortic dimensions," Grant replied immediately.

Beckett didn't need to look at the test for this; he knew the answer to be correct.

"What about question fifty-four?" Beckett asked.

Again, Grant looked off to one side before replying.

"What structures are most commonly affected by Vogt–Koyanagi–Harada disease?"

Beckett confirmed that this was correct.

"And the—"

Grant didn't even wait for him to finish.

"Bilateral, diffuse uveitis."

Who the fuck is this guy? Beckett wondered. *Doogie Howser?*

It was possible that Grant had managed to obtain a copy of the test beforehand; after all, Beckett put so little stock in these things that he usually just kept them stored locally on his hard drive. He also recycled tests year on year.

"And this memory of yours... does it work for everything?"

Grant shook his head.

"No. Only for medical-related topics. I think... I think I got it from my father."

Chapter 29

BECKETT HAD GONE FROM planning Grant's death one moment to being genuinely curious about the man in the next. But that didn't make it any easier to dial back his urge.

And this frightened Beckett.

Sure, he'd seen the man's eyes… Grant had a secret — *another* secret — of that Beckett was certain.

But that wasn't enough. Not *nearly* enough.

Was I really going to pull the scalpel out? he wondered. *Was I really going to kill Grant right here in my office?*

The rational part of his brain told him that that was ridiculous, that like with Wilson Trent and the others he needed solid proof that they had committed murder — he needed them to say it. But his lizard brain was still firing, and his fingers were still tingling something fierce.

Calm down, Beckett. Figure out if this whole eidetic memory thing is a sleight of hand, a red herring. Don't be rash; be calculated. Be safe.

He swallowed hard and interlaced his fingers on top of his desk, squeezing them tightly as he did.

"Why don't you tell me about him?" Beckett began, trying his best to stall. "About your father, I mean?"

Grant took his time before he answered.

"My dad was a good man and an even better surgeon. But growing up… he just didn't have much time for us. Often, when I was young, he'd leave me alone in his office while he was out working back to backs in residency. I'd have nothing to do but look at medical textbooks for hours on end. But I quickly ran out of material… I discovered that all I had to do was read a book once to remember everything within," Beckett paused. "He spoke about you, by the way."

This last part took Beckett by surprise.

He'd met Peter McEwing on several occasions; he'd even spent an entire month with the man on rotation during his residency. But that was more than a decade ago. It seemed improbable that Peter remembered him, unless, of course, he shared his son's alleged memory.

"Yeah? And what did he say about me, Grant? All good things, I hope."

Grant cleared his throat.

"He said... he said that you were different. That you weren't like the others, that you weren't an egocentric physician that had been forced into the profession by his folks."

Beckett raised an eyebrow.

"He said this?"

Grant nodded.

"He and a colleague used to talk about you."

"Flattery will get you... everywhere. Who was the colleague?"

Grant shrugged.

"I don't remember."

Beckett tried to maintain his composure. If Grant was indeed the person responsible for putting the organs on his desk, he was weaving one hell of an intricate yarn to cover his tracks.

What had started out as Beckett trying to grill Grant, to tease out if he was like the others, had turned into an ego-pumping affair about a late surgeon who was twenty years his senior.

And it was damn confusing... all of it.

But that didn't change the fact that Grant was still holding back, that he had a secret.

"Grant, your dad died from liver cancer, is that correct?"

"Yes. He was diagnosed with stage IV liver cancer that quickly spread to his bones and eventually to his brain and heart. He was dead within six months."

Grant's tone was strangely flat and even, unlike when he was recounting the other parts of the story. Whatever Grant was, it was clear that he loved his father.

But patriarchal endearment wouldn't save the man if he'd done what Beckett thought he had.

Nothing would.

"And there was no chance for a transplant? Replace his liver before the cancer spread?"

Grant replied in the same monotone voice.

"No. He wasn't a candidate. Can I… can I go now? I'm not feeling well."

Beckett nodded and watched Grant leave his office, more confused than when the man had first arrived.

Sure, Grant had a secret, but did he have a motive?

If Peter McEwing had been a candidate for a liver transplant but didn't get one, then Beckett could imagine Grant taking his frustration out on others. It was far-fetched, certainly, but given that their family name was plastered above a state-of-the-art transplant facility, it was in the very least understandable.

But both Beckett and Grant knew that a person with stage IV liver cancer would never be a candidate.

Beckett's phone buzzed on his desk and he quickly answered it.

"Dr. Campbell?" a screechy voice said.

"Lab Guy? What's up?"

"I managed—" he lowered his voice before continuing. "I finished the DNA testing on the two hearts that you gave me. What do you want me to do with the results?"

Beckett's eyes drifted to his computer. He was opposed to a paper trail but heading back to the lab for a second time was apt to raise eyebrows.

"Email them to me. And then incinerate both organs."

"Sure thing… and about that recommendation, do you think—"

"Yeah, yeah; I'm on it," Beckett said as he hung up the phone.

Shaking his head, Beckett opened the email that Delores had sent him, one that consisted of several video files. The first showed the hallway leading to his office with a timestamp from just after seven the day prior—not from the most recent delivery, but the second one. The second heart. About a minute in, a hooded figure suddenly appeared on the screen and Beckett felt his respiratory rate increase. Although the camera only showed the back of the man's dark outfit, the posture was obviously that of a man's. And tucked beneath his arm was a familiar-looking cardboard box.

"I've got you," Beckett whispered as he opened the second video.

This one proved less helpful, as it only showed a quick glimpse of the man's dark hoodie as he passed through the frame.

But halfway through the third video, the hooded figure turned and looked directly at the camera.

The glimpse only lasted a split-second, but it seemed like an eternity to Beckett, given that his breathing had stopped entirely.

Chapter 30

BECKETT WATCHED THE VIDEO several more times, freezing the image of the person who had brought the organ to his office several times, just to be absolutely certain.

There was no mistaking who it was.

And yet, Beckett was having a hard time believing it.

It wasn't so much *who* he had seen, but the underlying implications.

"It can't be," he said under his breath. "There's no fucking way."

And yet it *was*. The video proof was right there, right on his desktop computer.

"I thought I could trust you," he whispered under his breath.

A new email notification popped up and Beckett instinctively opened it, minimizing the video.

As he'd instructed, the content of Lab Guy's email was sparse and ambiguous. But the attachments were anything but: two DNA profiles, one from each of the most recent hearts that had been left on his desk.

Even though he knew the identity of the man who had dropped off the organs, it wasn't enough. Beckett still needed concrete proof that he had actually killed the people and removed their hearts, not just desecrated a couple of corpses.

Many people did bad things, things that required retribution. But Beckett's brand of punishment was reserved for only one specific act.

Murder.

He picked up his phone and dialed Detective Dunbar's number.

I know what you are. I know what you did.

"Dunbar, it's Beckett... Dr. Beckett Campbell. I've got one more favor to ask."

There was an uncomfortable pause and Beckett wondered if he was overstepping.

"What do you need, Beckett?"

"Listen, I've got some John Does—two of them—both dead and I'm trying to figure out everything I can about them before I sign off on their cause of death. I need their medical history, but I don't even have their names. Think you can help me out?"

There was another pause during which Beckett heard the man typing away furiously at his computer.

"Are they recent? I don't see any records of homicides in the system from the last few days."

"No, not homicides," Beckett lied. "Most likely accidental deaths. But I need to be sure... using them as a test for new residents, which is why I need their medical history. I managed to convince the lab to get me a couple of DNA profiles. The thing is, I still can't find their names. Think you can run the profiles through CODIS or missing persons?"

"Missing persons and accidental deaths... this isn't really my department," Dunbar replied.

Fuck.

Beckett debated pushing the man but decided against it. Dunbar already knew too much for his liking.

"I understand. Thanks anyway."

"Wait a second—just wait. What is this really about? I don't hear from you since... the *incident*... and now you call about car accidents and missing persons? What's going on?"

Beckett swallowed hard.

"Nothing, I just—"

"Is this," Dunbar lowered his voice. "Is this about what happened with Drake and the mayor... the *club*?"

And there it was; Dunbar himself had just given Beckett an out.

He cleared his throat.

"I can't... I can't reveal confidential information, as I'm sure you understand, Dunbar," Beckett said. "But... hypothetically speaking, this might be related to something bigger."

This wasn't a lie—not exactly. There *was* something bigger going on here, and despite how much he loathed the idea, Beckett found himself in the middle of it.

Again.

His own words repeated in his mind then, some of the last ones that he remembered saying to his friend Damien Drake.

No matter how hard you try to do the right thing, you just end up dragging everyone into the mud with you. Everyone, from Jasmine to Clay, to me, to Screech, you pull us all down.

Beckett couldn't help feeling like he was doing the same thing...

"Yeah, sure, I get it. Send me the profiles and I'll see what I can do. No promises, but I do understand the sensitive nature of the request," Dunbar replied at last.

Chapter 31

SUZAN CALLED A HALF-DOZEN times, but Beckett just let it ring out.

For once, he was indecisive as to what to do next. The last thing he wanted to do was to rush things, as he'd almost done with Grant, and make a mistake that he'd never been able to live with.

As for the person on the video, he'd have to wait until the cover of darkness to act on that.

But Beckett needed to do something… he needed to clear his mind for a few hours. As he saw it, his options were twofold: he could go to the bar and get drunk, ask Ron to join him—the man wouldn't need convincing—or he could see if any of the junior medical examiners needed his help.

He would much rather do the former, but if Beckett wanted to reclaim his status as the go-to Senior Medical Examiner, then he had to put in some face time. Besides, he had a favor he needed to return and there was no time like the present.

With a labored sigh, Beckett logged into the Medical Examiners portal. There were four active cases, two of which were suicides, while one was a gunshot homicide, and the other one was unknown. But he wasn't looking for a particular case, he was looking for a particular Medical Examiner.

And, as luck would have it, in the column listing the MEs name beside the case where the cause of death was still listed as 'unknown,' he saw *Karen Nordmeyer*.

Beckett clicked on the small clipboard icon to access more detailed notes.

The subject was an eighty-four-year-old man by the name of Armand Armatridge, if he could believe it. He had lacerations on his scalp and the police report stated that he'd been found in a pool of blood at the bottom of a staircase. It seemed cut and dry to Beckett, but it had already been fourteen hours and Karen had yet to sign off on the case.

Beckett packed up his things and made his way out of the office. As he passed Delores's desk, he felt a heaviness in his chest.

He hated the way he'd acted toward her, the way she now looked at him with fear in her eyes.

"Chris Hemsworth?" Beckett asked. "You sure?"

Delores looked momentarily confused but then nodded.

"Yeah… why are you asking me this?"

"No reason," Beckett said as he continued past.

***

Karen Nordmeyer looked up when Beckett entered the morgue. She was a mousy woman, with small features and brown hair that fell to her shoulders. Short, stocky, but intuitive and smart.

"Dr. Campbell," she said in a curious manner that was equal parts question, statement, and accusation.

"Dr. Nordmeyer," Beckett replied, doing his best to impersonate her tone.

"Did I… did I make a mistake? Is this about the Winston Trent case? Was I—"

Beckett shook his head.

"No, you did great—thank you for closing it as quickly as you did. The media… fucking vultures, I tell ya. If you had hesitated on reporting the cause of death as a suicide, you'd have spent the next year or so answering questions. Trust me on this one."

Karen nodded, but the look of confusion remained on her face.

"Are you missing a report, or…"

Beckett slipped on a pair of latex gloves.

"Nope, I was just bored and decided to swing by to see if you needed a hand. You know, returning the favor."

Confusion became relief—for *both* of them.

It appeared as if not everyone in the ME community hated Beckett, or feared him, after what had happened with Craig Sloan.

Beckett walked over to the body and stared down at the nude octogenarian.

"Thank God, because I can use all the help I can get on this one," Karen said.

Chapter 32

KAREN WAS RIGHT; THIS was a more difficult case than Beckett had first thought. And it only became more confusing when she shared the crime scene photographs with him.

In most of them, eighty-one-year-old Armand Armatridge lay at the bottom of the stairs, his feet extending into the hallway, his neck and head resting on the second to last step. This wasn't terribly unusual, but the sheer volume of blood was.

It was smeared on the walls, on the final few stairs, and pooled about his head in a viscous puddle.

"I've already shaved his head," Karen said, indicating the top of the man's skull. "As you can see, there are seven long incisions—but it looks like at least two of them are from a single impact."

Beckett craned his neck to get a better look.

There were indeed seven incisions, each one of them was four- to five-inches long, deep enough to reveal bone beneath. They were long and deep but weren't perfectly straight; they seemed to have a natural curve to them, Beckett noted.

"What about blunt force trauma?" he asked, even though he was fairly certain he knew the answer already.

"None; no evidence of subdural hemorrhage."

Beckett held the photograph from the crime scene close to his face, paying close attention to the individual stairs. In total, there were maybe fifteen or sixteen of them—it was tough to tell for certain, based on the angle of the image—but there only appeared to be blood on the bottom three or four.

"He definitely died from blood loss, there's no question about that. But the thing I don't get is why there's no blood on the stairs near the top. I mean, even if he did a somersault off the top landing, the first impact would have been no more than halfway down," Karen said.

"If he fell from the top, I would expect blunt force injuries to his skull and brain," Beckett informed her.

"Yeah… but we can't rule it out entirely. I mean, look at the wounds, see how they're curved?"

Beckett nodded.

"I see that, but they are most definitely from the stairs."

"But rounded like that?"

"Yep. A round object moving perpendicular to a flat edge—such as the edge of a stair—will give the impression that they were caused by a curved object."

"Huh. Didn't know that. But the blood? Why only at the bottom? If he fell down the stairs like his wife who found him claimed…"

Beckett chewed the inside of his lip.

"The wife said that? That he fell *down* the stairs?"

Karen grabbed a folder off the table beside them and opened it. Then she started to read the statement.

"Wife made her way back inside after an evening out on the porch, only to find her husband at the bottom of the stairs. She couldn't tell if he was breathing and immediately called 911," Karen flipped to another page. "Ah, here it is, in the 911 call: *Please, my husband… he fell down the stairs and there's so much blood… you need to send someone…*"

"Well, that's just not true."

Karen put the piece of paper down and looked at him, eyebrow raised.

"He didn't fall down the stairs? How can you tell?"

Beckett walked around the man's body and pointed at a small scuff mark on his chin. Then he used two fingers to pry open his mouth and ran them along his bottom teeth. Beckett doubted that they were Mr. Armatridge's real teeth, but that didn't matter; they were rough enough to nearly cut his gloves.

"Because the first impact was on his chin—there is no way that happens if he fell down the stairs. I bet that you'll find a small, corresponding dot of blood on the seventh or eighth step. He hit his chin hard enough to chip her bottom teeth and then he flew *backward*. So, he hit his chin on stair eight, say, and then fell backward. Based on his height—five feet nine, maybe—the next point of contact would be near where his head came to rest. That's why you don't see any blood on any of the top steps."

Karen seemed impressed.

"So, he fell *up* the stairs, not *down*. But it could still just be an accident. I mean, his wife was distraught and people say fell down the stairs all the time, irrespective of the direction of the fall."

Beckett didn't answer right away. Instead, he rolled the man onto his side and stared at his back. Then he palpated the flesh beside his spine.

"This was no accident. Feel here," he instructed.

Karen did as she was told, using her own gloved hands to prod the dead man's flesh.

"I don't—" she suddenly retracted her hands, her eyes going wide. "His ribs… they're broken."

"Yeah, and if you wait another day or so, you'll see some bruising that will look suspiciously like handprints."

Beckett's phone buzzed and he tore off one of his gloves and pulled it out of his pocket.

"So, he was pushed then… but that can't be right."

Beckett looked at his phone. It was Detective Dunbar.

"Why's that?" Beckett asked as he made his way toward the door.

"Because his wife ... Beckett, Mr. Armatridge's wife is wheelchair-bound."

Now was Beckett's turn to be surprised.

"Well, then I guess there was someone else there after all," Beckett said as he opened the door. "'Twas the one-armed man, *mon cheri*."

Chapter 33

"DUNBAR, TELL ME YOU'VE got something?" Beckett walked briskly as he spoke, heading toward his office.

"Well, I plugged your DNA profiles into the system and… uh, Beckett?"

Beckett nodded at a doctor in a white coat who passed and lowered his voice.

"Yeah? What is it?"

He half expected Dunbar to say that the match came from victims from the Second World War. Only that didn't make sense, because the organs were still fresh.

"I was just wondering, is what I tell you covered under doctor-patient confidentiality or something? Because…" he let his sentence trail off.

Beckett rolled his eyes. Not only was Dunbar not his patient, but the information wasn't even about him. It didn't matter, anyway; in reality, there was only one type of confidentiality that would hold up in court: lawyer-patient confidentiality. In the medical world, court-ordered injunctions often broke sealed hospital records.

"You don't need to give me names, Dunbar. Just tell me what you can about these people, if they are missing or not… just enough so that I can construct a proper medical history."

"Okay, but still—you didn't get this from me, alright?"

"Sure."

Beckett's mind was already racing, wondering what could be so damning. After all, they were on the same side, weren't they?

Dunbar cleared his throat and continued.

"Well, Subject A—let's just call them subjects from now on—was released from juvie just two weeks ago. Spent three years there for robbing a convenience store and beating the owner nearly to death."

Beckett's eyes narrowed as he took this in.

"What about Subject Two or B or whatever?"

"Subject B was older but was also just released from a two-year stint for possession with the intent to distribute. Heroin."

Beckett inhaled sharply.

Two young, recently released criminals killed by unknown means, their organs were subsequently harvested and sent to my desk, he thought.

Beckett didn't care much for coincidences and didn't think that the similarities between the victims were random.

Two criminals, both—

Something in his mind clicked.

"Dunbar," he said, his voice barely a whisper. "When these criminals were released, were they sent to a halfway house of sorts?"

Dunbar made a *hmph* sound. It was clear that they were heading into deeper waters here, water that Dunbar wasn't so much concerned about wading through as he was drowning in.

Beckett didn't blame the man. After all, despite the fact that they knew each other fairly well and were most definitely on the same side when it came to most things, Beckett knew that his reputation had changed over the last little while.

Not everyone in the NYPD had come to the same conclusion as Internal Affairs when it came to Craig Sloan's demise.

"Okay, fine. I get it. Let me just ask you this… if they were released at the same time, what are the chances they were released to the same halfway house? Even if one wasn't technically a juvie."

"There's a strong possibility."

"And would this particular place happen to be called—" Beckett cursed himself for not being able to remember names. "—the New York Renewed Life House?"

He cringed; the name wasn't exact, he knew that but hoped that it was close enough that Dunbar caught his meaning.

Dunbar said nothing. Normally, this would have been good enough for Beckett. But he'd almost jumped the gun earlier and wasn't about to make the same mistake again.

"Dunbar, you don't have to answer. Sometimes, when you don't answer, it can be interpreted as a 'yes,'" Beckett said slowly. "For the purpose of my residency class, were Subjects A and B both released to the NYC Renewed Life Halfway House?"

Beckett let the dead air extend for ten seconds before nodding.

"Thanks, Dunbar, I owe you one."

Beckett hung up the phone and then looked around. He was halfway to his office now, but he'd had a change of heart.

He wasn't going there anymore. No, Beckett suddenly had more pressing matters to attend to.

Chapter 34

FUCK OFF, SUZAN, BECKETT thought as he looked at her number that lit up his cell phone. He didn't know how many times she'd called during the day—at least a dozen—but he'd refrained from answering a single one of them.

The truth was, Beckett wasn't sure he could trust her anymore.

Not after her supposed 'friend' had broken into his house.

Not after the same man had been released to the halfway house that Beckett currently sat outside of in his car, waiting for the sun to finally go down.

Not after he'd seen Brent Taylor's face, as clear as the day was long, carrying the cardboard box to his office on video.

Beckett had indulged on some greasy fast food between going home to collect supplies and making his way to the halfway house, the remnants of which were on the floor of the passenger seat.

And now, he'd resigned himself to watch people come and go, waiting for one, or maybe two, people in particular.

It wasn't enough for him to just take out those responsible for removing and delivering the organs; Beckett had to find out what the man had on him, and if Suzan really was involved.

I know what you are. I know what you did.

"Yeah, and I know what the Fuck you are, too," he grumbled.

Beckett glanced at the passenger seat, his eyes falling on the leather case lying on it. Inside were some rudimentary lock-picking tools, two new scalpels, as well as several syringes. Only, this time, they weren't just filled with midazolam but a mixture of midazolam and the powerful paralytic agent succinylcholine.

He'd opted for the same style tracksuit as he'd worn for his encounter with Winston Trent but had forgone the saran wrap beneath. It was simply too hot and restrictive. Besides, with all the riffraff he'd already seen come and go outside the halfway house, in the rare event that he left some DNA behind, it would be just one of hundreds of samples.

And, worst-case scenario that there was a match with his profile from the Craig Sloan incident, he had a reason for it being there: he'd had an altercation with Brent Taylor at his house and Grant McEwing had been in his office that very day.

Beckett reached for his balaclava and, with gloved hands, turned it into a hat. It was an eclectic look, one that would have normally been out of place during a warm late summer evening, but based on what he had already seen, everything from a Paperbag Princess to man in a tux, he thought he fit right in.

His phone rang again.

Take a Hint, Suzan.

Beckett exhaled deeply and let it go to voicemail.

His mind drifted as he waited, and Beckett found himself wondering if he'd filled the ink from his home tattoo kit since Winston Trent.

He thought he had, which was good. Good, because he had a feeling he might be adding another tattoo to his collection very shortly.

Beckett leaned back and closed his eyes for a moment.

The last few days had taken more out of him than he'd initially realized. The lack of sleep didn't help, either.

But all that would change.

Based on prior experience, he knew that after he ended this, his reward would be one full, uninterrupted night of sleep.

Beckett had no doubt that the nightmares would come later, but not tonight.

Not after he killed Grant McEwing.

Even though it had been Brent's face on the recording, Beckett had already come face-to-face with the man.

There was no way that Brent had the skill, or the foresight, to remove a liver and put it on dry ice.

No, he may have been the messenger, but the eidetic freak, Grant, was behind all of this.

Beckett grimaced.

And maybe Suzan.

The thought sent a shudder up his spine.

Beckett heard a couple talking and slowly opened his eyes.

A couple, dressed in nice but not ostentatious clothing, approached the front of the halfway house. There was a young man leaning against the wall near the entrance—he'd been there for the last half hour or so, chain-smoking—who seemed oblivious to everything except for his cigarettes. But when he saw the couple, he flicked his cigarette away and stood up straight.

Beckett leaned closer to the windshield and tried to get a glimpse of the newcomer's faces.

And then, just as smoking man reached for the door and pulled it wide, the couple turned.

Beckett smiled.

He'd been right all along; it *was* Grant.

Grant McEwing was responsible for murdering those kids.

Beckett took one final deep breath and then grabbed the leather case from the passenger seat and tucked it into the inside pocket of his sweatshirt. He was about to step out of his car when he saw someone else start to approach the still open door.

Someone else he recognized.

The smile immediately sloughed off his face.

"No, it can't be. *Please.*"

PART III

Halfway Home

Chapter 35

GRANT AND SUZAN… THEY'RE working together, Beckett thought.

Is the same thought that he'd had a dozen times already, one that he just couldn't shake.

Twice he had stepped out of his car, only to get back in again. Their partnership made sense, in a sick way.

I know what you are.

Suzan most definitely knew about him, about what he was. He didn't think that she knew all the details, but maybe she was just referring to what had happened Craig Sloan.

I know what you did.

Well, Suzan knew that, too. She knew that Beckett had brained Craig Sloan, bashed his skull in with a rock until he was dead. She couldn't have known about the way his fingers tingled afterward, the overwhelming sense of euphoria that embraced his entire being, but she didn't have to.

The author of the notes had only said that they knew what he'd done and what he was.

What Beckett had done was killed, which made him a killer.

Sure, he had his rules, his moral code, but he was still a killer.

And while Suzan might not know about the others—about Ray Reynolds, Donnie DiMarco, Bob Bumacher, Boris Brackovich, and Winston Trent—you only needed one notch in your belt to be labeled a killer.

"Fuck," Beckett said through gritted teeth. He still didn't understand her connection to Grant McEwing or the reason why they're putting organs on his desk.

And he couldn't fathom Suzan actually committing murder. Sure, she was snarky and feisty, but a murderer?

Beckett knew killers; he'd stared into Winston Trent's eyes less than a week ago.

He also looked in the mirror every day since.

Neither Grant nor Suzan shared the same, blank stare, the empty eyes.

But the evidence...

Not today, Beckett thought. *Not now. Go home, get some rest. You can't make a mistake, not with the stakes this high. Not when it comes to Suzan.*

After what felt like hours of deliberation, but couldn't have been more than ten minutes since Suzan had followed Grant and his date into the halfway house, Beckett put his leather case back in the glovebox.

Then he started his car and drove home.

***

To Beckett's dismay, Suzan's appearance at the halfway house wasn't the final surprise of the night.

There was a man seated on the stoop of Beckett's house when he pulled into the driveway.

"Can I help you?" he asked.

The man raised his head and held a bottle of Scotch out to Beckett.

"I promise that it wasn't opened when I got here... but hell, Beckett, you work so damn late, I just had to dig into it."

Working... that's one way of looking at it.

Beckett didn't feel like a social call, not now, but it was clear that the man had been waiting for a while.

"Ron, you alright?"

Ron shrugged and Beckett got a good look at him in the light for the first time. He wished he hadn't asked; Ron definitely didn't look 'alright.' He was pale and clammy.

And judging by the reek of alcohol coming off him in waves, he was drunk to boot.

"Never mind, don't answer that. You want to come in for a drink?"

Ron offered a weak smiled and then used the railing to haul himself to his feet. He grunted so loudly that Beckett immediately went to his friend to lend a hand only to be shooed away.

"I thought you'd never ask," Ron said between labored breaths.

Chapter 36

"YOU LOOK INTO THAT thing that I asked you about?" Beckett said as he peeled off his sweatshirt and tossed it onto the couch. He took one whiff of the armpit of the T-shirt beneath and recoiled.

It smelled rank.

He got a fresh one from the top drawer of his dresser.

"I did, actually. Looks like your pal Dr. Singh picked it up and slapped a UNOS number on it. I'm thinking that it's found a new home in someone very deserving. Maybe even someone famous."

Beckett, who was in the process of removing his shirt, paused.

"Famous, huh?"

Ron chuckled.

"Maybe, who knows."

Beckett smiled despite himself.

Maybe even Chris Hemsworth. Wouldn't that be ironic? Wouldn't have a problem setting Delores up if that were the case.

Ron extended a finger with glass in hand toward Beckett's side as he put on his T-shirt.

"New tattoos?"

Beckett glanced down at the horizontal lines beneath his arm and then quickly pulled his shirt down.

"Did them myself. Trying to work up the courage for something a little more elaborate."

Ron sipped his Scotch.

"Well, keep practicing."

Beckett took the bottle of Scotch off the table and poured himself a glass. He drank greedily, barely tasting the liquid as it rolled aver his tongue. Knowing Ron's taste, he expected it to be something cheap and powerful.

He wasn't disappointed.

"I can't believe you drink this shit," Beckett said under his breath. Then he raised his eyes to look at Ron once more. In the bright lights of his home, Beckett realized that Ron wasn't just sickly looking, but he looked terrible. His eyes were sunken, his cheeks sallow. "In fact, I don't think you should be drinking much at all."

"Yeah, I'm feeling a little under the weather these days. But it'll pass; it always does."

Beckett considered this for a moment.

"These things pass... until they don't; until the last one."

"Thanks, Aristotle," Ron replied with a chuckle.

"I consider myself more of a Socrates Marxist, to be honest," Beckett shot back, choking down another sip.

Despite the kerosene-like flavor, or maybe because of it, the alcohol was doing its job. And, as was always the case, the two men spoke more freely with every subsequent drink.

"Hey, I heard a rumor that some of your students aren't that happy with you."

Beckett shrugged.

"What else is new. They're used to being coddled, to being given a textbook that they can regurgitate to pass a test. Forensic pathology isn't like that; there are no cut-and-dry answers. Every case is different, every one requires them to use their measly brains to solve. But try telling that to Dr. Hollenbeck."

Ron laughed.

"Well, that's exactly who I heard it from, in fact. Dr. Hollenbeck was muttering to himself when he came to see you at your office, something about abusing your students. Speaking of which, you have the McEwing kid in your class?"

The mention of Grant triggered something in Beckett and he took a moment to answer.

"Yeah, he's one of my R-1s. He's... a different cat."

Ron leaned in close.

"How so?"

This time when Beckett's eyes narrowed, they stayed that way.

"He's got an incredible memory... Why are you so interested in the McEwing kid?"

Ron leaned back and sipped his drink.

"Funding... it's always about funding. In addition to procuring your lost liver, it looks like Dr. Singh is making some inquiries about funding for the new transplant wing. Boring shit, to tell you the truth."

Beckett recalled his meeting with Dr. Singh and the way the man had been so candid about the funding issues.

"What about the funding?"

Ron shrugged.

"You're on the board, aren't you?"

"What do you want me to do about it?"

"Rumor has it that more funding is coming the Unit's way, enough to actually get the doors open. I'm thinking that maybe you can steer the McEwing kid in another direction, just for a little bit."

It took a moment for Beckett to clue into what Ron was saying.

"...so that Dr. Singh looks like an asshole for the whole ribbon-cutting ceremony when the place stays closed. And, maybe—just *maybe*—they start to look for a new director?"

Ron smiled and raised his glass.

"I knew you were special even back when you were a budding young medical student."

Beckett finished his drink and placed the empty glass on the table.

"I'll see what I can do. Now, I don't mean to be a dick, but I'm tired as hell—and it looks like we can both use some rest. What do you say?"

I'm thinking that Grant McEwing is going to have more to worry about than funding in the near future, Beckett thought.

Ron picked up the bottle and tilted it onto its side. Then he emptied the contents, splitting it between both glasses.

"One for the road?"

Chapter 37

"SUZAN... SUZAAAAAAN... WAKE UP, Suzan."

Beckett stared down at Suzan's face, the slackness of her jaw, her slightly open mouth, the relaxed skin around her eyes.

She stirred and Beckett leaned forward. As he did, moonlight reflected off the scalpel in his hand.

"Suzaaaaan..."

The woman's eyes snapped open and she looked up at Beckett, a startled expression on her face.

Instinct took over and she tried to move, tried to sit up.

Only she couldn't.

Suzan pressed her chin against her chest and Beckett followed her eyes. He stared at the heavy leather belts that secured both her legs and arms to the bed.

Her eyes flicked back up to his.

"Beckett? What are you doing? What's going on?"

Beckett swallowed hard.

"Why am I tied up? Why are you holding that... Beckett, what the hell is going on?"

Beckett averted his gaze; he couldn't stare at her any longer without tears forming in his own eyes.

He looked down at her body, at the lacy bra that covered her breasts, her white underwear. She was in great shape, but the moonlight gave her goose-pimpled flesh an odd hue.

Blue... like that of a corpse.

"Beckett? Why are you doing this?"

Even as he brought the scalpel close to her wrist, Beckett couldn't look at her face. Suzan's hand tightened into a fist, but the bindings held fast.

"Why?" she pleaded.

"*Because,*" *Beckett said as he pressed the scalpel against her skin, drawing a thin red line of blood. "Because you killed, Suzan. And now you have to pay.*"

Chapter 38

BECKETT AWOKE SOAKED IN sweat. The sheets were so damp that when he tried to press himself up onto his elbows, he slipped back down onto his pillow.

He closed his eyes and then immediately opened them again when he saw Suzan's face staring back.

"Please," he said into the darkness. His tongue was thick and he felt lightheaded as he always did when he drank too much the night prior. Or was it still the night of?

Beckett turned his head to the clock on the bedside table. The glowing green numbers read 5:35.

Traditionally not much of a morning person, or an early riser, Beckett had found himself waking earlier and earlier each day. As a result, he'd been relegated to only a few hours of fitful sleep every night.

But that was the beautiful thing about the human body; it could adapt to a great number of different scenarios, be they environmental are self-imposed stresses.

But the mind... the mind wasn't nearly as plastic as the body.

With a groan, Beckett managed to sit up and then waited for the world to stop spinning. When this sensation subsided, he made his way to his bathroom and chugged a glass of lukewarm water.

It wasn't just the nightmares that were keeping him up at night, the terrified faces of his victims that appeared in his sleep. It was also the sheer gravity of what he'd done.

Taking a person's life, no matter how much they deserved to die, changed you in ways that were irreversible.

And yet, that wasn't the worst part; the worst part was the expectation—no the *need* to do it again that was nearly crippling.

"Fuck," he grumbled as he peeled off his drenched T-shirt and boxers and stepped into the shower.

Tonight, Beckett thought. *I have to take care of this tonight if I ever want to sleep soundly again.*

***

A hot coffee and a bagel with butter later, Beckett started to feel little better. The passage of time, no matter how small, also helped.

He parked in his spot outside NYU medical and then walked inside, keeping his head low.

Once inside the building, several colleagues said hello, but Beckett stemmed potential conversation by keeping his head low. He didn't feel like speaking to anyone.

The only person he couldn't pass without engaging was Delores.

"Morning," he said, raising his coffee cup in mock salute.

Delores nodded, clearly still sour from the way that he'd unfairly berated her.

"Dr. Hollenbeck was looking for you," she said curtly.

Beckett scratched his head.

"Does he ever sleep—do you, for that matter?"

He'd meant this as a joke, but Delores wasn't buying it. She pressed her lips together tightly.

"I could ask you the same thing."

Beckett nodded.

"I wish I could," he said as he started down the hallway toward his office.

"Dr. Campbell?"

Beckett turned.

"Yeah?"

"There's a student waiting for you in your office."

Beckett felt his lip curl and his heart start to race.

He didn't feel in the mood to speak to anybody, least of all Grant McEwing. They'd chat soon enough, but not now. Now he had to keep up appearances. Now he had to get ready for class so that people didn't notice anything out of the ordinary... *more* out of the ordinary.

He debated turning and leaving just then, going straight to his class even though it didn't start for another hour, but figured that that would raise further suspicion.

There were just too many threads out there, too many things that pointed directly at him should anything sinister befall Grant.

With a sigh, he thanked Delores again.

"FYI, Suzan's in your office, too. And she didn't seem... *herself.*"

Beckett stopped cold.

"S-S-Suzan... Suzan's in there with him?"

Delores eyed him curiously.

"Not with him... with *her.*"

Chapter 39

"**WHAT CAN I DO** for you?" Beckett said as he entered his office. While he was grateful that Grant wasn't the student in question, he would have picked the McEwing kid over Suzan in a heartbeat.

Suzan, tied to the bed, dressed only in her underwear.

"Why are you doing this, Beckett?"

Maria glanced up at him, a scowl on her face.

"It's not fair," the woman began like a petulant child.

Beckett frowned. He loved teaching, but he hated babysitting.

"What else is new," he grumbled.

Suzan, the expression on her face matching his own, glared at him.

"What happened to your phone?" she demanded. It became clear at that moment that her being here had nothing to do with Maria.

She was here to see him.

Beckett averted his eyes—he couldn't bear to look at her, knowing what she'd done.

Keep it together, Beckett. You can't afford to make any mistakes.

"Dropped in the shitter this morning after taking a dump," he said, looking instead at Maria as he spoke.

The woman's eyelids retracted to their maximum as Beckett deliberately stepped between Suzan and Maria, and then squatted on his haunches.

"I'm sorry, please, tell me what your problem is."

Clearly confused by the room dynamic, Maria took a moment to collect her bearings.

"I just don't think it's fair... you don't teach us anything on the first day and then on the second, you give us a final exam? I wasn't ready! I have a very specific routine that I go through before every test I take, and because the final was such a surprise, I didn't get to do any of it. I think... I think that this significantly affected my performance."

Beckett stared at the woman as if she were a five-year-old instead of in her mid-twenties.

"You know what? I think you're right."

Beckett turned to Suzan and snapped his fingers before pointing at the pile of tests on his desk.

"Suzan, doll, would you be so kind as to pass me Maria's test?"

Suzan's scowl became a sneer, but she did as he asked and handed it over.

"All right, Maria, let's see here," Beckett looked down at the paper in his hands. He tried to keep a straight face, but when he saw how poorly she'd done, he faltered for a moment. "Suzan, the red pen, please?"

Suzan threw it at him and he barely managed to grab it after it bounced off his chest.

Beckett added a zero after the ten percent she'd scored, then turned the page for Maria to see. With a placating smile, he said, "Problem solved. Congratulations, you aced this one!"

Again, that same bug-eyed expression.

How does she get into one of the most exclusive residency programs in the state and scores ten percent on an exam that a first-year med student could at least pass? Is this her first introduction to pathology? Shit, to anatomy? To medicine?

Something inside Beckett's head suddenly clicked.

If Grant was behind all of this, then this wasn't his first crime. Nobody goes straight from parking tickets to murder and organ removal.

Somewhere... somewhere there's a record of other, minor crimes. Of a pattern of escalation.

Beckett realized that with Suzan in the room with him, he was trying to rationalize his way out of what was to come.

But that wasn't a bad thing... was it?

"Is this... is this a trick?" Maria asked.

Beckett shook his head and held the test out to her.

"Here, take it."

Maria hesitated but eventually grabbed the paper.

"Good. So that settles it... so that's fair, right?" Maria raised a manicured eyebrow expectantly. "I'm sure that if I poll all of the other residents, that they'd agree, no?"

Maria opened her mouth to say something, but no words came out.

"Yeah, I think in this morning's class I'm going to ask them just how they feel about it—about you going from ten percent to a hundred just by whining. *That's* fair. I mean, you come in here, in my office—actually, you went to Dr. Hollenbeck first, didn't you?"

Maria just gaped.

"Of course, you did," Beckett continued. "Because that's fair, too. It's fair for you to go directly to the head of the department, rather than coming to speak to me first. So, we'll just see what your fellow residents have to say."

"You wouldn't," Maria gasped.

Beckett held his hands up defensively.

"Why not? Lemme guess... that's *not* fair?"

Chapter 40

WHEN THEY WERE FINALLY alone in his office, Suzan glared at Beckett.

"Seriously, Beckett, what in God's name is your problem?"

Beckett did his best to avoid her eyes. In his mind, he erected a wall, separating the old Suzan from this new version.

"What? No witty come back? No snarky remarks? What the hell is going on with you, Beckett?"

Beckett could hold his tongue no longer.

"What's wrong with *me*? Care to tell me where you were last night, Suzan?"

Now it was Suzan's turn to avert her gaze.

"I was out."

"Yeah, no kidding you were out—I saw you. I saw you at the god damn halfway house."

Suzan's eyes shot up then, once again boring into his soul.

"You *followed* me?"

Beckett started to shake his head, to tell her that he was going there anyway, but then changed his mind. That would be a difficult one to explain.

"Yeah, you did—sure you did. But do you want to know why I was there?"

Beckett tempered his excitement. Yes, he very much wanted to know why she was there. Except he doubted that the next words out of her mouth were going to be the truth.

"Because I was looking for my friend, for Brent. The man that you threw out of your house, the man who had nowhere else to go. *That's* what I was doing."

Beckett raised an eyebrow.

"You sure about that, Suzan? You sure that's why you were *really* there?"

Suzan bolted to her feet so quickly that her chair nearly toppled.

"What are you saying, Beckett? What are you getting at?"

"Are you sure you didn't go there to see Grant?"

Suzan's face sucked inward.

"Who the fuck is Grant?"

"Oh, okay, so now you're going to pretend like you don't know him, like you weren't standing beside me during the ribbon-cutting ceremony for the transplant unit that has his name on it."

"Grant *McEwing*? Now you've really lost your mind."

"Yeah, I saw him there, too. Arrived just a few minutes before you, in fact."

Suzan opened her mouth to say something, but then closed it again. After a short pause, she finally spoke, only this time, her voice was unnaturally calm.

"You *were* spying on me," she accused.

"I was just—"

Suzan suddenly stormed past him.

"You know what? I'm fucking done with this. Get someone else to mark your tests. I quit."

Beckett felt a mixture of emotions then, sadness, but also relief.

"That's what you wanted, right? A way out?" Suzan spat as she reached for the door handle. As she pulled it wide, she turned back one last time. "By the way, you've got another delivery. You can deal with that one by yourself, just like everything else. Because that's the way you work, right? Keep everything to yourself. Beckett and his little fucking secrets."

Chapter 41

BECKETT STOOD FROZEN IN the center of his office long after Suzan was gone.

Eventually, his phone buzzed on his desk and this drew him out of his near catatonic state. He walked over to it, but instead of answering, he bent and looked beneath the desk.

He thought he was prepared for what was beneath, but he wasn't.

It was another box with the exact same dimensions as the three previous packages.

For some reason, Beckett had thought because he'd figured out who was sending them, that the packages would stop coming.

Clearly, this was not the case.

Three days, three different packages.

Breathing in shallow bursts, Beckett picked up the package and put it on his desk. Only, this time he didn't open it; he just stared at it.

Suzan and Grant were becoming more brazen; shit, she'd even pointed it out to him.

Beckett shook his head repeatedly, trying to wrap his mind around what was happening.

It was a mistake to go to sleep last night, he realized. It was a mistake go to sleep without taking care of the problem. And because he had, another person was dead.

Making up his mind, Beckett picked up the box and started towards the door. As he made his way down the hallway, he tried his best to regulate his breathing.

"Delores, you wouldn't happen to know who delivered this parcel today, would you? I'm getting sick and tired of people sending me flowers, seeing as I'm allergic."

He sounded like a robot, but it was the best he could do given the circumstances.

"I'm sorry Dr. Campbell, but I was delayed this morning. If you really want to know who delivered it, I can get you the security footage again," she hesitated before adding. "And, by the way, I'm not allergic, so…"

"Yeah, please send me the video. As for the flowers, trust me, these aren't your type. They're full of bugs."

***

Beckett sat alone in his lab, which was roughly the size of a large cubicle that was fully enclosed with an opaque door. There was a computer on the desk, typically reserved to print requisition forms, as well as all the tools a pathologist needed to process specimens.

And that's what he was, at that moment; Beckett was no longer a killer, no longer someone desperately searching for the person who sent him the organs, but a pathologist.

He sliced open the box on the table in front of him and folded back the cardboard. As expected, in addition to the white transplant bag inside, he found a note on yellow paper: *ONE BEAT, TWO BEAT, THREE 'PEAT.*

Beckett's upper lip curled, and he debated putting the note on the scanner to decipher the hidden message as he'd done before. In the end, he decided against it.

He was done with riddles and puzzles.

Instead, Beckett opened the vinyl bag and stared down at another human heart.

After removing it from the plastic biohazard bag, he picked
it up with both hands and held it up to the light. Based on the
size and color—it was a dark pink and lacked any overlying
fat—it was apparently from another young person. He turned
it in his hand, examining the precision by which it had been
removed. The cuts weren't perfect for a transplant; the aorta
was slightly too long and the pulmonary artery too short. The
superior vena cava, perhaps the most difficult vessel for an
unskilled hand to remove, was jagged, reminding him of
hesitation marks.

Beckett frowned.

He'd hoped that there was something in this newest
delivery that would rule out Suzan and Grant—he was still
holding onto the fleeting idea that he'd made a mistake about
their involvement.

But the cuts were consistent with those of a second-year
medical student. As for Grant, he'd had more training, more
experience with autopsies. In fact—

Beckett's back straightened.

The autopsy!

Beckett replaced the heart in the bag first, and then put that
inside the transplant cooler. Then he removed his gloves and
bolted from the lab.

Chapter 42

"**OUT! EVERYONE OUT!**" **BECKETT** shouted as he entered the morgue. A junior ME named John Knox turned to look at him. When he saw who had entered, he pulled the mask off his nose and mouth.

"Excuse me?"

Beckett frowned.

"I need the room for ten minutes. Out!" he repeated. Standing beside John was a woman that Beckett didn't recognize.

The woman turned and looked at John expectantly, and act that only served to infuriate Beckett further. Sullied reputation or not, he was still the Senior ME here.

"I said, *get out!*"

For a split second, it looked like John was going to refuse, but he eventually decided better of it and slammed the locker with the cadaver he was inspecting closed. As he made his way toward Beckett, he gestured for the woman to follow.

"It's only a matter of time, Beckett," John whispered in his ear as he passed.

Beckett scowled and bit his tongue.

It's only a matter of time before I fucking choke the life out of you, he thought.

After John and his minion had left the room, Beckett hurried over to the row of lockers near the back. He scanned the names taped to the exterior and eventually found what he was looking for: lockers identified by the name 'Forensic Pathology' further labeled with numbers R1 through R8.

These contained the cadavers that Beckett had used on the first day of class, the ones that the residents had been tasked with determining the cause of death.

He racked his brain and recalled that Grant McEwing had had the second body, one that he'd correctly diagnosed with liver failure.

Beckett grabbed the locker handle with R-2 on it and opened it. A fan clicked off and cool air rushed towards him. Then he yanked out the tray that the cadaver lay on.

The man's flesh was paler than it had been when Grant had cut him open, which was to be expected given that he'd spend two days in the locker. His rib cage as still open, but the skin flaps from the Y-incision had been folded back like a poorly wrapped gift.

Beckett slipped on a pair of gloves and then slowly peeled back the man's skin. He was obese and it took some effort to pull the thick blanket of yellow fat back to reveal the body cavity beneath. As expected, the organs had been replaced after Grant had determine the cause of death.

Crinkling his nose against the smell—the cooling process and the fan could only do so much—Beckett reached inside the body and pulled out the heart.

It was much larger than the one in his lab and covered in fat, but that's where the differences ended.

Like the special delivery, the aorta was too long and the pulmonary artery too short.

But these could easily be chalked up to inexperience, mistakes that even a junior transplant resident might make. But when he turned the heart over, he saw something that was unique: hesitation marks on the superior vena cava.

This was a surgical signature if Beckett had ever seen one.

"I've got you now," he whispered to the dead.

Chapter 43

AFTER REPLACING THE HEART in the cadaver's chest and closing the locker, Beckett hurried back to his lab. He was more certain now than ever that Grant McEwing was the one sending him the organs, and the one removing them, but he still didn't know *why*.

As for the notes… they had to be Suzan's doing—that was the only thing that made sense. But what was the connection between them?

Was it just the fact that she knew Brent Taylor and he was released to the halfway house funded by the McEwing Foundation?

But that didn't make sense… the timing would have had to have been perfect, given that the first organs—the liver and heart—were delivered on the day Brent was released.

That was too… *coincidental*.

Beckett pulled open the door to his lab and stepped inside. He started towards his computer when his eyes fell on his desk.

His *empty* desk.

Beckett turned around briefly to confirm that this was indeed his lab.

It was.

"What the fuck? What the fuck happened to the cooler?"

His heart started to race again and he looked out into the hallway. There was no one to be found in either direction.

"What the hell is going on?"

Was it John? Did he come in and steal the goddamn organ?

Beckett re-entered his office and blinked several times, trying to will the cooler back into existence. But it wasn't there. His tools were still laid out as he had left them, but the entire bag—even the box—was missing.

Beckett, grasping at straws now, got on all fours and looked beneath the desk.

Nothing.

He threw his hands up in frustration.

What the fuck!

Rising to his feet again, Beckett searched the entire lab for the box, knowing that if it wasn't on the desk where he'd left it, it wasn't there at all, but he was unable to help himself.

After a minute, Becket gave.

It was just another thread linking him to these crimes that he would have to wind up later.

Right now, however, he needed to find a link between Suzan and Grant that predated Brent's release from prison.

Pulling up to his computer, he did a quick search on Grant McEwing. This was the easy part; the man had a press release dedicated to him following the ribbon-cutting ceremony.

Grant McEwing, brother to Flo-Anne and son to the late Peter McEwing and long deceased Mary Beth McEwing, is a twenty-five-year-old recent graduate from McGill Medical School in Montreal, Quebec.

Beckett drummed his fingers on the desk but stopped when it didn't sound right with one digit missing.

McGill… McGill… who do I know at McGill?

Beckett snapped his fingers, which was also awkward without a full-length middle finger.

Diego!

Another quick search and Beckett found his old residency buddy's phone number.

"Diego!" he exclaimed when the man answered, trying to push the fatigue and everything else from his mind.

"Yes, this is Dr. Diego Lopez. Who's this?"

"*Tsk, tsk, tsk.* Diego, you're supposed to go from waif to coquettish, not the other way around. Everyone knows that."

He could almost hear his friend smile on the and then the line.

"Dr. Beckett Campbell, the only tatted up pathologist that I know who drives a motorcycle."

"Yeah, just another pretty face. How are you? Still recovering from our night out in Montréal?"

"I'm always just recovering from a night out in Montréal."

"Good point. How are ya?"

"Living the dream," Diego replied. "Last time we spoke, you tricked me into telling you about one of my patients. I'm assuming you want something similar this time? After all, you are a needy bastard."

"What can I say, I'm an only child," Beckett said with a chuckle. "Only this time, I don't need to know about a patient, but a student."

"Really? This about that young girl you sent up here to do an internship a while back?"

Beckett shook his head.

"No, it's about a medical student. His name is—wait, what girl? Girls I tend to remember, names, not so much."

"You said it was a favor for a cop buddy or something. Suzanne or Suzan Cuthbert or something like that. Jesus, Beckett you need to stay off the booze. Beckett? Earth to Beckett?"

Beckett's mouth hung open.

Now that Diego mentioned it, he *did* remember sending Suzan to Montréal when he first heard she was interested in medicine a number of years back. As a favor to Drake.

And that's the connection, he thought, his heart sinking into the pit of his stomach.

"Beckett? You still there?"

Beckett was still on the phone, but his mouth was suddenly so dry that it felt as if he'd swallowed a handful of cotton balls.

"Yeah," he managed to croak. "I'm still here."

"What's the name of the student you want to know about?"

Again, Beckett struggled to swallow.

"Grant McEwing; he was a medical student—graduated the year before last."

"Never heard of him."

Beckett started to strum his fingers again.

"You sure? He's got this freaky memory, possibly eidetic."

"I don't know the name, but I can ask around if you want."

What Beckett wanted was to get out of this nightmare. What he wanted was to never receive a random heart on his desk in the first place.

What he wanted was for Suzan *not* to be involved.

"Okay, thanks. Appreciate it, Diego."

"No problem. Let me know when you're back in Montréal so we can get together again."

"Sounds like a plan. Take care, Diego."

Beckett hung up the phone and then collapsed in his chair.

Chapter 44

THE ONLY THING THAT kept Beckett going was the knowledge that if he didn't act now, tomorrow morning there'd be another delivery waiting for him.

Which mean that there'd been another murder.

Tonight, he had to take out Grant. After that, he would figure out what to do with Suzan.

On the way out of the morgue, he passed by the main lab, inside of which he spotted the junior ME, John Knox, sidling up to the woman who was with him earlier.

Without thinking, Beckett opened the door and leaned inside.

"John, if you don't put the fucking box back on my desk by the time I come in tomorrow, you're not gonna work another day as an ME in New York."

John whipped around.

"What? What the hell are you talking about?"

Beckett seethed.

"One day; you have one day to put the box back."

With that, Beckett slammed the door closed hard enough to rattle it on its hinges. As he continued down the hallway, he spotted someone coming toward him.

"Ron?" Beckett said, confusion washing over him. It certainly looked like Ron with skin the color and texture of wax paper and sunken eyes.

The man smiled as Beckett approached, his thin lips stretching and cracking. It was indeed Ron.

"Beckett, just the man I was looking for. I heard it on the grapevine that Dr. Hollenbeck is looking for you. Apparently, you missed class today? Beckett, I'm feeling a little bit like your mother, here."

Beckett had completely forgotten about class and Dr. Hollenbeck.

"Thanks, man. But I'm busy right now... can we chat later?" he asked as he walked by Ron.

The man gave him a curious look but nodded.

"No problem. But the next time I see you, you better have a bottle of Scotch in your hand. You owe me."

"Sure thing," Beckett said as he left the morgue.

***

As darkness descended on New York City, Beckett found himself back at the halfway house. It was busier today, which bode well for him; easier to get lost in the crowd.

He kept his eyes trained on the door for several hours, and eventually, like yesterday, Grant returned. And once again, he was accompanied by a woman that Beckett didn't recognize in the dim light.

He waited for them to enter and then stepped out of the car and followed.

Smoking man was there again, perched against the wall, a fresh cigarette dangling from between his lips.

Beckett tilted his head downward as he grabbed the front door and entered the *New York City Renewed Life Center*.

The first thing that struck him was the smell. Based on the clientele, Beckett half expected the place to reek of body odor and urine, but he was pleasantly surprised.

It smelled clean—not hospital clean, but sanitary even though he thought he detected the scent of meatballs being fried somewhere to his left.

The main entrance hall that Beckett found himself in held several rows of metal tables that reminded him of his high school days.

Glancing around to catch his bearings, he noticed that the walls were mostly bare, aside from a cluster of photographs of smiling youths.

Those who made it out… alive, Beckett thought morbidly.

Beckett tucked his gloved hands into the front pocket of his sweatshirt and kept his head low as he passed a group of tattooed teenagers who were discussing last night's Yankee game.

Looking up only long enough to confirm that neither Grant nor his partner was in this main room, he hurried toward a set of doors that had just swung closed off to the left.

The thick, double doors were marked *Longterm Only,* whatever that meant, but nobody appeared to care, or even notice, as Beckett walked toward them. They were unlocked, and Beckett opened one of them just wide enough to step through.

Rather than another room, the doors led to a staircase that extended in both directions. Below, Beckett spotted a red door that looked like it might lead to a boiler room of sorts. There was a second door beside the red one—also marked *Employees Only*—but this one had a thick padlock that would be nearly impossible to break.

Up it is, he thought, as he started to ascend. On the second step, he spotted a colorful pamphlet and bent to pick it up.

On the front was an image of the *New York City Renewed Life Center,* beneath which was a slogan written in bold type.

Home is where the heart is.

A smile crept onto Beckett's lips as he hoisted himself up the stairs.

Yes, Grant was definitely guilty. Guilty of murder. And like the others—like Craig Sloan and Donnie DiMarco, Ray Reynolds, Bob Bumacher, Boris Brackovich, and Winston Trent—he was going to pay.

As Beckett took the final stairs that led to another door, this one, like the double doors, marked with the words *Longterm Only*, he felt his fingers start to tingle with a familiar feeling.

Chapter 45

LONGTERM ONLY EVIDENTLY REFERRED to sleeping quarters, but if it were up to Beckett, he might have dubbed them *Jail Cells*.

On either side of a long hallway that doubled-back over top of the main room below, were small, cell-like rooms containing just a table and a cot. The doors were made of some sort of Plexiglass, but they were so stained by greasy smudges that looking through them had a sort of funhouse effect.

And this is what they have to look forward to after *they're released from prison*, Beckett thought.

He hurried past these rooms, his head still bowed. Most were unoccupied, but the few people he witnessed were either sleeping or engrossed in a game of cards with other shady-looking characters.

Beckett kept his focus trained on the door at the end, the one marked *Employees Only*. When he reached it, however, he was dismayed to find it locked. But after what had happened with Bob Bumacher, after nearly being strangled to death by the white hulk, he'd come prepared.

Beckett teased a small, lock-picking device from the leather case. The halfway house was old, as were the locks on the doors. After just a few seconds of playing with the locking device in the old tumbler lock, he heard the pins line up and the mechanism disengage.

He slid the device back into his pocket, looked around once more to confirm that he was alone, and then pulled the door open.

Beckett's intention had been to quickly and discretely slip inside this room as he had the others, but he stopped short.

It was as if he'd opened the door to some sort of portal.

He was looking into an immaculately kept office that seemed so out of place in the dingy hallway, that he actually peered back to confirm that what he was seeing was real.

The desk facing the door was made of granite or some other precious stone, and on top of it rested a brand-new laptop computer. The desk lamp alone looked like it cost three figures, and that said nothing of the ornate pencil holder beside it.

"Well, this is interesting," Beckett muttered as he stepped inside and closed the door behind him.

On either wall behind the desk, were two other doors.

Beckett went to the one on the left first. There was a rectangular window embedded in the wooden door and he peered through. The inside was nearly identical to the *Longterm* quarters in the hallway, only there was no cot. Instead, there was a large table that took up most of the room.

Beckett didn't need to see the leather straps on each corner to know what that table was for; four men had lost their hearts on that very surface.

"Tsk, tsk, tsk," Beckett said up under his breath. "You've got a nice set up here, Grant."

He pulled the handle, only to find the door locked. But instead of trying his hand at picking it, he turned his attention to the other door in the room. Unlike the first, this one had no window—it was a solid hunk of blue metal—which was more intriguing.

But Beckett's enthusiasm was short-lived; it was securely fastened by a new padlock. After trying unsuccessfully to pop it open with his tool, he gave up and took a step backward, looking for another way in. The hinges were thick and sturdy, but with the right equipment, Beckett thought that he would have no problem removing the entire door.

But he hadn't come prepared with an entire toolbox; he only had his rudimentary lock-picking device and his killing implements.

I could come back...

Beckett immediately vanquished the idea.

Last time he'd decided to 'come back' another kid from the halfway house had lost his life.

I'm not leaving here without Grant McEwing's heart in my hand.

Just as he came to this conclusion, Beckett heard the door behind him start to open.

Chapter 46

"**Dr. Campbell?**" **Grant McEwing** gasped. "What are you… what are you doing here?"

Beckett was equally as surprised to see Grant but recovered quickly. He instinctively reached into his pocket and grabbed the lock-picking tool and squeezing it in his palm. He preferred his scalpel, but the new blades were still tucked away in the leather case.

Beckett reached out and grabbed Grant by the collar and pressed the lock-picking tool against the man's throat before he even knew what was happening.

"Hey!" Grant shouted as the door closed behind him.

"I know what you did," Beckett hissed in his ear as he backed Grant up against the desk. He was staring directly into Grant's eyes as he spoke.

"What are you talking about?"

Beckett didn't say anything; he just readjusted his grip on the man's collar and squeezed tightly. When it became clear that Grant wasn't going to put up a fight, he released the man but kept the lock-pick at the ready.

"I'm here… you called me out, and now I'm here. *I know what you did. I know what you are.*"

Beckett expected Grant's eyes to harden then, to acquire the steely stare of a killer that he'd only been able to identify once he'd committed the act himself.

But it never came.

Beckett grabbed Grant's collar again, this time pulling him forward until their faces were but inches apart.

"*I know what you did,*" Beckett accused again.

And then, Grant's eyes *did* change, but not in the way that Beckett expected.

Inexplicably, they softened.

"Okay, okay," Grant said in a quiet voice. Beckett relaxed his grip but didn't let go completely. "It's true. It's all true."

His eyes started to water and Beckett leaned away.

This was not how he'd expected the man to react once confronted; after all, the hidden messages made it clear that he *wanted* Beckett to know who he was.

What he'd done.

But this… this was just confusing.

Or maybe it's a ruse, Beckett thought as he slowly reached inside his pocket to retrieve the leather case.

"What did they do? What did they do to deserve to die?" Beckett demanded.

Grants eyes suddenly whipped up and focused on Beckett's.

"*Die?* What are you talking about? I just… I just lied on my forensic pathology application. I didn't even go to medical school."

Beckett was so stunned by this response that he took a step backward.

"You *what?*"

"Yeah, I know it was wrong and probably illegal, but I never went to medical school."

Beckett's eyes bulged.

"What the fuck are you talking about?"

"I faked the transcripts, said I went to school in Montréal. Got a friend of my dad's to write me a recommendation letter."

Beckett shook his head.

"But… but that room," he said under his breath, indicating the door with the window just behind Grant.

"This isn't even my office," Grant replied quickly.

Beckett's mind was swimming now.

It *had* to be Grant.

He was the one who knew Suzan, the one who started residency the day this all began. Grant was at the ribbon-cutting ceremony, he was part of the foundation that funded this place… all things pointed at him as being the one who'd killed those kids.

And the cuts… the cuts on the heart were the same.

"It's not?" Beckett asked in a strangled tone he didn't recognize.

Grant shook his head.

"No… it's my sister's."

Chapter 47

"YOUR... YOUR SISTER?" BECKETT stammered, moving further away from Grant.

"Flo-Ann," Grant said with a nod. "This is *her* office."

Beckett was reeling now. He remembered seeing her at the ceremony a few days prior and —

An image of Grant entering the halfway house with a woman at his side flashed in his mind.

Was that... was that *her*? Could it have been her all along?

"Did she... did Flo-Ann go to medical school?" Beckett asked.

Grant nodded.

"But only for two years... I helped her every way I could, and when I couldn't, dad stepped in. She just wasn't... cut out for it."

Beckett was floored.

That explained why the cuts were the same; Grant never had any formal training. What he'd learned in textbooks, he'd taught his sister. It made sense that their cuts would be nearly identical.

And that was also why Grant didn't have the look in his eyes of the other killers—because he wasn't one.

"Are you going to kick me out of the University? Call the cops?" Grant asked.

Beckett had to think about this for a moment, he had to go over everything he'd just said to Grant.

Did I implicate myself?

In the end, it didn't matter; despite the potential consequences, Beckett was unwilling to break his moral code and hurt this kid, even if it meant saving himself.

"Get out of here," Beckett hissed, deliberately avoiding the question. "Get out of here, now!"

Grant took a moment to react, but when he did, he bolted for the door.

But before he left, Beckett thought of something.

"The keys… do you have the keys to this room?" he asked, pointing to thick blue one to the right.

Grant nodded and pulled a keyring out of his pocket.

"Give it to me," he instructed.

The frightened man tossed the keys at Beckett and he caught them.

"Now leave!"

Grants, who looked like a deer caught in headlights, sprinted out of the room.

When he was alone again, Beckett made his way over to the thick metal door and started trying the keys one by one. On the fourth or fifth try, the padlock unlocked.

After a deep breath, Beckett opened the door.

The first thing that struck him was the smell; the room reeked like meat left out on a hot summer day. The second thing he noticed was the buzz of the flies.

Blinking to clear his vision, Beckett finally caught a glimpse of what was behind door number two.

And then he gasped.

Beckett was no stranger to death; and yet, the scene before him took his breath away.

There, at the back of the room covered haphazardly with a blue tarp was the outlines of three bodies. Whoever had covered them had done such a poor job that Beckett could make out a clump of dark brown hair matted with blood poking out of one corner. Holding his breath now, Beckett strode over to the tarp and pulled it back with one sharp yank.

Then he staggered, slipped on some indiscernible slime, and fell on his ass.

There weren't three bodies beneath, but four.

And he recognized the fourth.

The man's mouth was open, frozen in fear, and his eyes were milked over. It was a snapshot of terror that shocked Beckett to his core.

It was Brent Taylor, the man who had broken into his house, Suzan's friend who she claimed had hit his head in high school.

The same man that Beckett had pushed away.

It dawned on him then that Suzan might not be involved in any of this after all. If Grant lied about going to med school, and Diego couldn't remember him, there was likely no connection between the two. And Beckett couldn't fathom her doing something like this to her friend, especially not after their interaction back at his house.

Flo-Ann must have come across Brent and convinced the simple man to help her, to bring the boxes to his office. And then she had either grown sick of him, or she was worried that he would give her up and had made him her fourth victim.

But if the fourth heart I received was Brent's, then who brought that one to my office?

Before he could think this over, however, Beckett heard the sound of footsteps approaching from down the hall. These weren't the sounds of running shoes; these were high heels.

Still on his ass, Beckett scooted across the slippery floor, breathing through his mouth to avoid the stench of rotting flesh. And then he did the only thing he could think of at that moment. He curled up next to Brent's ravaged body and pulled the tarp on top of them.

Then Beckett waited.

Chapter 48

THE STENCH WAS SO bad beneath the tarp that Beckett's eyes started to water. He could hear the heels as they clacked on the hard cement ground when the woman entered the room, but then they stopped. Beckett assumed that Flo-Ann had just noticed that her kill room door was open.

As subtly as possible, he reached into his pocket and pulled out the leather case. Then, working blindly, he managed to tease out a pre-loaded syringe. As he adjusted his first and third fingers on the guards—something he was still getting used to without his middle finger—Flo-Ann muttered a curse under her breath.

A second later, he heard the clacks as she approached the blue door.

The pressure in the room suddenly changed and some of the reek of death wafted out as the door was pulled wide.

Beckett held his breath and waited as the slow clacks came closer… and closer… and closer…

The movement stopped and, after a short pause, he heard the tarp crinkling as someone seized a corner.

Unlike how he'd yanked the tarp, Flo-Ann peeled it back slowly, gradually revealing Beckett's smiling face.

Flo-Ann's pretty face went white and she tried to retreat to the door. But her heels slipped and she fell to the ground much like Beckett had minutes earlier.

That's when Beckett lunged, leading with the syringe. Flo-Ann didn't even get her hands up before he injected her in the side of the neck.

"I know what you are," he whispered in her ear as she started to struggle beneath him. *"I know what you did."*

Chapter 49

BECKETT STOOD OVER TOP of Flo-Ann's body as her eyes slowly fluttered and then eventually opened.

A characteristic look of confusion washed over her pretty features, but these eventually turned into a sneer. She tried to sit up, but the best she could do was move her head.

Her eyes drifted to the leather straps that held her arms out to her sides and then the ones that spread her legs. Beckett had stripped to her bra and underwear, and when she realized this, her face transitioned from a sneer to a smile.

"Nice set up you have here," Beckett said, looking about the room.

It was almost fitting that he killed her here, in the same room that she'd taken the lives of the four recently paroled men and young boys.

"Why can't I move?" Flo-Ann asked.

Beckett held up the half-empty syringe.

"*Succinylcholine*," he said. "The perfect killing drug. I only injected half the required dose, mind you; not enough to paralyze your heart or diaphragm. Only your muscles."

Even though Flo-Ann had the cold eyes of a killer, Beckett still needed her to say it. He needed her to say that she had killed those men and boys before he went through with it.

Beckett picked up a scalpel and held it up to the incandescent lights above. It reflected harshly on Flo-Ann's face.

"Why did you kill them, Flo-Ann?" Beckett asked in an almost bored tone.

The sneer returned.

"My dad was a good man... no, a *great* man. What he did for others, including the people in this halfway house and the people he saved as a surgeon? He deserved better. But when he needed help, when he needed a new liver, you think that he could get one?"

Beckett listened intently, waiting for the confession he needed to hear.

"He was on the donor list for six months, but by the time his name popped up, he was as good as dead. The cancer had spread to his heart and his brain. He was reduced to a bumbling idiot unable to wipe his own ass, let alone save anybody."

Beckett bit his tongue. This was a common refrain among socio- and psychopaths like Flo-Ann; they justified their actions any way they could. But even if Peter McEwing had died from old-age at 103, Flo-Ann would have found another reason to kill.

Beckett knew this because he felt the same urge.

His fingers were tingling so intensely now that he could barely hold the scalpel steady. His face was flushed and sweat started to break out on his brow.

"You know why I sent the organs to you, Beckett?"

Beckett shook his head and leaned forward. He placed the scalpel on Flo-Ann's skin, just below where her collarbone met her shoulder.

"I'm listening."

"Because you're like me," she said. Beckett started to slide the blade into her flesh, reveling in the way that it cut through the connective tissue as easily as a hot knife through butter. Flo-Ann didn't even notice; the succinylcholine had numbed her entirely.

For now.

"I'm not like you," Beckett replied in a flat affect.

He pushed the blade deeper and moved it to the center of her chest.

"Oh, yes you are. It was only an accident that I saw you outside of Winston Trent's house—just an accident. I don't even usually go to that neighborhood, but I was following one of the juvenile delinquents that my dad saved, who was stealing from the halfway house."

Beckett drew the scalpel to her belly button, splitting her flesh and leaving a trail of blood behind. Then he started again from her opposite shoulder, completing the Y-incision.

"I couldn't believe it at first. In fact, I wouldn't have even have recognized you if you weren't on the board of directors for the McEwing Transplant Unit. So that's why I sent the organs to you because I knew you were like me. We can work together, we can—"

Flo-Ann's eyes suddenly fluttered and rolled back as blood spilled out of the Y-incision and coated her alabaster flesh.

Beckett was amazed that she hadn't yet clued into what was going on.

"We can still... work... together..."

he woman grunted as Beckett peeled her skin back and then moaned when he cracked her sternum. Not only was Flo-Ann's kill room well-equipped to remove organs, but Beckett had even found one of the organ transplant bags that she'd stolen from the McEwan Transplant Unit.

As he reached inside her body cavity, her mouth opened and blood spilled onto her cheeks.

And yet, she didn't scream, which Beckett assumed was partly from the paralytic and partly because she knew that this was coming. She *must* have known that it was destined to end like this.

"You're... like... me..." Flo-Ann managed between coughs and spatters of blood.

Beckett worked quickly now, knowing that with the amount of blood she was losing, it would only be a matter of time before she died.

But unlike Flo-Ann, Beckett had training—considerably more than just two years of medical school.

As he reached inside Flo-Ann's chest cavity and finally pulled her heart free, he held it up for the woman to see a second before her eyes rolled back in her head. Then, covered in the woman's blood, Beckett leaned close to her ear.

"You and I are nothing alike."

Chapter 50

BECKETT SHOWERED WITH HIS clothes on first, cleansing himself of any of Flo-Anne's DNA, before putting them in a bag while still in the shower. Then he scrubbed himself with antiseptic soap as if he were a surgeon preparing to operate.

Then he tied up the bag and left it in the tub. He would incinerate it later back at the lab.

After drying off, Beckett went to his bedside table and pulled out a black leather attaché case. Only this one wasn't filled with syringes or scalpels, but a homemade tattoo kit.

With a deep breath, he prepared the ink and then lifted his right arm. As he stared at the six lines that were already, Beckett recited the names they represented.

"Craig Sloan, Donnie DiMarco, Ray Reynolds, Bob Bumacher, Boris Brackovich, Winston Trent."

And then, with a characteristic wince, he started to tattoo a new line, this time adding another name to his collection.

"Flo-Ann McEwing."

When he was done, Beckett placed saran wrap over the new tattoo.

Exhausted, he made his way back to his bed and, for the first time in a long time, ever since the night he'd killed Winston Trent, Beckett slept soundly and without nightmares.

***

"Morning, Delores," Beckett said with a grin. He sipped his coffee and then put another cup on the woman's desk.

Delores looked at him with a curious expression.

"What's this?" she asked.

"Extra tall mocha one pump with cream, just the way you like it," he replied with a wink.

Delores stared at them as if he had three heads.

"Oh, and you know Chris Hemsworth? Because I do," he said. "Well, not really. Last time he was here filming in town one of the directors came to me to fix a problem... crabs, you know how it is. Anyways, as luck would have it he's in town tonight for a gala and he brought Chris with him. I called in a favor and put your name on the guest list."

Delores blinked several times and Beckett thought for a moment that she might pass out.

"I really am sorry about the other day, Delores," Beckett said, his tone turning serious. "Anyways, why don't you take the rest the day off and get you saw something pretty to wear for tonight."

With that, Beckett turned and started toward his office.

"Dr. Campbell?"

"Yes?"

"I got footage from the hallway the other day, just as you asked," Delores said, holding a USB key out to him.

Beckett frowned and took it.

"Thanks," he replied hesitantly and made his way to his office.

Beckett took a seat behind his computer and loaded the video.

Halfway through, his coffee cup slipped from his hand and spilled to the floor.

"No fucking way."

Chapter 51

BECKETT WAITED IN THE dark. At around 9:30, the door opened and a light flicked on.

The man who entered dropped his briefcase and then made his way toward the kitchen. Halfway there, he spotted Beckett sitting comfortably in his lounge chair, an expensive bottle of Scotch clutched in one hand.

"I see you brought the bottle you promised me," Dr. Ron Stransky said, a smile on his face.

Beckett rose to his feet and held the bottle out to him.

"Better than that swill you drink," he said.

Ron nodded and started to say something, before his eyes drifted to the other item that Beckett had brought with him to the man's house.

"Is this what I think it is?" Ron asked as he stared at the white vinyl bag.

"Yeah."

"I figured as much," Ron said. "I figured that it would come down to this."

Beckett still said nothing even as he walked over to his old friend and lifted the hem of his shirt. Beneath, he saw a large section of gauze that covered most of the right part of his stomach.

"All those years of drinking caught up to you, didn't they?"

Ron nodded.

"I've lived a good life, Beckett. I won't deny that. And I won't make any excuses."

It was a curious choice of words, and Beckett let them sink in for a moment.

"It wasn't hard to find someone like Flo-Ann to help me out," Ron continued. "But she just couldn't control herself. One liver, I said. Just one. To be honest, if you hadn't taken her out when you did, then I probably would have."

Beckett slowly took the scalpel out of his pocket. He prepared himself in case Ron started to run or tried to fight him, but the man didn't even flinch; he was too frail from his recent liver transplant.

Beckett didn't have to look to hard to find out who had taken the liver from Lab Guy—it had been Ron.

Beckett couldn't believe that he'd fallen for Ron's story about Dr. Singh coming to get it... the man was square as they came, worried about funding and protocol and all sorts of nonsense that didn't really matter at all.

"So, you coerced her, got Flo-Ann to do your bidding?"

Ron shrugged.

"You know as well as I do that if I didn't approach her, she'd find another reason to kill."

Beckett found himself nodding despite everything that had happened.

I can't believe I thought it was Grant when the entire time it was Flo-Ann.

The rest of the story clicked into place then. Beckett recalled how he'd asked Grant who his father had been speaking about Beckett with. At the time, Grant had said he didn't remember. But that was Grant's thing: remembering. He didn't want to tell Beckett, because it had been Ron all along. And Ron had written the fake letter of support so that Grant would get into Beckett's residency program.

All of this begged the question of how long Ron had actually planned this—how long he knew what Beckett had done, who he was.

"Why me? I understand why you got Flo-Ann involved, but why me? Was it just that she saw me with Winston Trent."

Ron sighed and shook his head.

"You remember back in residency? The night that we are in the 'merge alone? There was supposed to be an attending there, but he'd left to screw one of the nurses. It was just you and me—remember?"

Beckett racked his brain but only managed to come up with a choppy recollection.

Ron nodded.

"The cops came that night, brought a man involved in a home invasion. But he wasn't a victim; he was the one who broke into the home and tried to abduct a seven-year-old girl. Remember that? The father shot him and the man in the 'merge returned fire. But while the father died at the scene, the intruder was brought to our hospital."

Images started flooding back now, filling Beckett's mind with stills of a man covered in blood, screaming that he was dying, that he'd been shot in the leg.

To... *please, God, save me! I don't want to die!*

"Yeah, I remember."

"I gave the case to you and took a supervisory role. It was a simple fix—fuse the femoral artery. Likely, he would have lost his leg, but he would have survived. But what did you do? You delayed, asking for more tests, citing nonsense about allergies or some other shit. Do you remember that?"

Beckett closed his eyes tightly and shook his head.

"I don't—I don't remember," he said.

"Well, I do. I'll never forget the day when you let a man bleed out right there on the operating table when you could have saved him. I'll never forget it because I saw something in your eyes then. That's when I learned what you were like—

what you were *really* like. I'm just surprised it took you so long to figure out for yourself."

A tear ran down Beckett's cheek as he raised the scalpel. Ron surprised by holding up a hand.

"I've made my peace, Beckett; I'm just hoping that you can allow me one last thing before you take my life."

Beckett lowered the blade a quarter inch.

"What?"

Ron's eyes flicked to the bottle in Beckett's hand.

"Just a drink—*one* drink. It's a shame to let that good stuff go to waist. Let me have one drink before it's all over."

Epilogue

"SUZAN? WHAT ARE YOU doing here?" Beckett asked.

Suzan was sitting on his porch steps, her face buried in her hands. When she pulled her face free, her eyes were raw and her cheeks were damp with tears.

Beckett ran to her then, wrapping his arms around her.

"What happened?"

Suzan didn't answer; instead, she grabbed the newspaper from beside her on the stoop and held it out to him. Beckett only needed to read the headline to know why she was crying.

On it, was a picture of a young Dr. Ron Stransky. The headline read: *Prestigious surgeon murders five—including a wealthy heiress—to harvest organs for himself.*

It was like something out of our novel.

Beckett's breath hitched.

"Brent... Brent was one of Dr. Stransky's victims," Suzan said between sobs. Beckett squeezed her even tighter. After several moments, she pushed him away and the rubbed her eyes.

"You care," she said in a whisper. "You pretend not to, but I know you care. You were there that night outside the halfway house because you care, because you were looking for him—for Brent—weren't you?"

Beckett stared at her pretty face, her soggy cheeks, before answering.

He nodded.

She was already broken; there was no point in destroying her completely.

Suzan nodded back and Beckett cradled her head in his arms.

After a few minutes, Beckett's phone buzzed in his pocket and he took it out.

It was a message from his friend Diego in Montréal.

No record of Grant McEwing ever attending medical school here, sorry bud. When you coming to visit, anyway?

"Who is it?" Suzan asked.

Beckett turned off his phone and slipped it back into his pocket.

"Nobody," he replied, pulling her to their feet. "Hey, how about we take the rest of the week off and go on a mini vacation?"

Suzan looked up at him with a knitted brow.

"I thought you hated vacations?"

"I hate the sun and the beach, but I love Montréal. What do you say?"

Suzan wrapped her arm around his waist. When her fingers brushed against his side, Beckett winced.

"I guess we should start packing, then. What's wrong with your side, anyway?"

Beckett started up the steps to his house.

"Nothing. Just got some new ink done—two new tattoos. Come on, let's go pack."

END

Author's Note

BECKETT IS ONE BAD *mamajama*. It was a lot of fun writing about his particular brand of vengeance, about his growth as a killer. It's not often that the killer is the protagonist in my book or any other, for that matter. So far, it's been a unique and satisfying journey and I hope you had as much fun reading it as I had writing it.

I have many more stories of Beckett and his growing gang of misfits—I'm thinking that Grant might stick around for a while, despite what happened to his sister—but I only have so much time to write them. That's why I insist that if you liked this book, then you leave a review on Amazon. This will help me gauge your interest in Beckett and his adventures and keep on writing them. With this series, Drake's Series, and Chase Adams's series, I have my hands full. Oh, and in case you didn't know, Beckett plays a prominent role in the Drake Series. My intention was to write **ORGAN DONOR** so that you don't *have* to read any of the other series to understand or enjoy it. That being said, if you dig Beckett, you might want to check out the Detective Damien Drake series.

…all this to say that there will definitely be at least one more book in Beckett's Series (although I would love nothing more than to write a couple dozen starring him). It's called **INJECTING FAITH** and involves Beckett traveling down south to confront a charlatan who has everyone convinced that he's performing medical miracles. Sign up to my newsletter or follow me on Amazon to get an update as soon as it goes live.

As always, you keep reading, and I'll keep writing.

Best,

Patrick

Montreal, 2018